Praise for Alan Davidson's
Body Brilliance

"*I love this book and you will too.* Body Brilliance *is one of the most enlightened— and enlightening—books I have ever had the privilege of reading. It reads like a memoir and is absolutely compelling, not to mention unique and practical; like a combination of Ram Dass and Christopher Isherwood.*"

— Krandall Kraus, Lambda Literary Award winning Author of *Bardo,* and *It's Never About What It's About: What We Learned About Living While Waiting To Die*

"*My little evangelical heart beat fast when I began to read Alan Davidson's* Body Brilliance. *Thanks to St. Paul, Augustine, and my grandmother, Noni, I learned at an early age that my body "was the enemy" and that I "should wage war against it." Then along comes Alan with another gospel altogether. What good news it is to learn again that our body is not just our friend but a powerful ally on our journey to spiritual wholeness. What an amazing book.*"

— Mel White, Co-founder of Soulforce and Author of *Stranger at the Gate*

"*Knowledge is power, to be sure, and Alan Davidson's superb new book,* Body Brilliance *demonstrates that knowledge may also be beauty—in the form of health, harmony, and multidimensional enlightenment. This book stands out from the crowded field of holistic and integrative books in that the author obviously possesses and is able to communicate, a depth of spirit and brilliance of intellect far eclipsing the average health care expert. With stunning photographs by the talented Victoria Davis, Davidson's exquisitely crafted style conveys a host of startling and wholly original revelations on the care and maintenance of the human body, mind, and spirit.*"

— Todd Michaels, M.D., Author of *The Twelve Conditions of a Miracle* and *The Evolution Angel*

"*Body Brilliance is a brilliant display of wisdom and beauty. It not only shares profound truths about the living body that everybody can use, but shows us, via Alan Davidson's personal journey, how real wisdom is born through honest seeking and perseverance. This is a lovely book. I hope its light shines everywhere.*"

— Robert K. Hall, M.D, Author of *Out of Nowhere,* Co-founder of Lomi School, Dharma teacher: www.eldharma.com

"This book chronicles one man's journey and transformation into the brilliance of embodied consciousness. It's a story of courage, passion, discipline, and joy; as well as being pragmatic, insightful, and educational. It's a beautiful book!!"

— Richard Strozzi-Heckler, Ph.D., Author of *The Anatomy of Change* and *In Search of the Warrior Spirit.*

"This book is a very personal homage to the miracle of the Human Body, and its God-given gifts to all of us. Learn how to Celebrate and Sing our 'Body Electric,' and Dance with Spirit. Let the Five Moving Forces of CHI shine through us, Being Fully Alive!"

— Chungliang Al Huang, Founder-Director, Living Tao Foundation, Author of *Embrace Tiger, Return To Mountain*

"Body Brilliance seamlessly integrates diverse modalities into practical solutions that everyone can apply to changes in their life."

— Dawn E. Clark, Author of *Gifts for the Soul*

"Wow! Body Brilliance is very well written and very honest. To that I would add passionate. It is truly an enjoyable book to read and I love all the autobiographical material. It certainly elevates the book from a treatise on the body to something filled with heart and soul. Great job!"

— John Collins, Sisters, OR

"I totally devoured Body Brilliance … skipping around some … but before I knew it I had read it all."

— Ann Lasater, Parthenon, AR

BODY

BRILLIANCE

WITHDRAWN

Mastering Your Five Vital Intelligences

by Alan Davidson

photography by Victoria Davis

www.BodyBrillianceBook.com

3 1257 01950 8059

Elite Books

Santa Rosa, CA 95403

www.EliteBooksOnline.com

Library of Congress Cataloging-in-Publication Data

Davidson, Alan

Body brilliance : mastering your five vital intelligences / by Alan Davidson ; photography by Victoria Davis. — 1st ed.

    p. cm.

Includes bibliographical references and index.

ISBN 1-60070-025- X

    1. Exercise—Psychological aspects. 2. Sports—Psychological aspects. 3 . Physical fitness—Psychological aspects. 4. Body, Human. 5. Mind and body. 6. Health. I. Title.

RA781.D363   2007

613.7'1—dc22

2006027107

Copyright © 2006, Alan Davidson

Cover design by Victoria Valentine

Typesetting by Karin Kinsey

Edited by Melissa Mower

Copyedited by Joanne Austin

Typeset in ITC Galliard

Printed in USA

First Edition

10 9 8 7 6 5 4 3 2 1

For my grandmother

Thelma Mayfield

for always, always believing in me.

Nanny, I love you as big as the sky.

CONTENTS

SECTION FOUR:
BODY WISDOM

ACKNOWLEDGMENTS

How do I begin to thank all the people who have helped to create this book? I gleaned the stories I share in these pages from a lifetime of learning, watching, listening, sharing, and loving.

Thank you to Nancy Winters for introducing me to bodywork as a spiritual practice; to Ann Lasater for teaching me, by her example, how deep that practice can go; and to Robert Hall, M.D., Richard Strozzi-Heckler, Ph.D., and the Lomi School for touching us all. Thanks also to David Lauterstein for his work in Deep Massage and to Terry Fritz for her work in polarity therapy.

Bless you, Victoria Davis. Your vision and talent have made *Body Brilliance* a work of beauty and art. Heartfelt appreciation to the six models who posed for these pictures: Kioka, your inner beauty is every bit as lovely as your body; Sean, Liza, Gabriel, Freddie, and Dawn, your strength and grace are amazing. Thank you Sarah Lipscomb for spending so many hours Photoshopping the images for print. Of course, the book would not be complete without Katie Ozanick's superb drawings, or Keith Belli's rendering of Leonardo da Vinci's Vitruvian Man, loaned to me by Carla Weebles; and David O. Hill's paintings (bless your soul, whatever realm of heaven you find yourself).

Special thanks to Greg Jeu, Jim Hurst, and *OutSmart Magazine* for believing in me and encouraging me to write, and to Ann Sieber and Joan Garbo for helping me find my voice as a writer and speaker. Thanks to Joanne Austin for her inspiration, for holding my hand, and for tirelessly editing and rewriting, and to Karla Eoff for editing as well. Leslie Walker provided writing tips and moral support, while Teresa Anderson generously shared her computer technical expertise.

Thank you to Hilary Smida, Mary Ann Foster, Patty Reed, and especially J. D. Arnold for taking the torch and carrying it forward. J. D. and I have shared so much of this journey together.

Much thanks go to Kathi Austin for sharing the laughs, the friendship, and her country house, and mucho amore to Rogers Adams for the lake house, the laptop computer, and for his love and support.

My heartfelt thanks to the Essential Touch regulars—Tom, Randy, Henry, Creighton, Michael, both Karens, Katy C., Darcy, Jack M., and John C.—for their confidence in me. I couldn't have made it without you.

Thank you to Jim Giulian for your quiet strength. You make loving fun.

DISCLAIMER

The principles and exercises described and illustrated in *Body Brilliance* are directed to people in overall good health. The opinions stated here are posed by a Texas state registered massage therapist and are not intended to replace the expertise of a licensed medical professional.

It is always wise to consult with your doctor or other medical professional before you begin any new health or exercise program.

Introduction

A life lived in fear is a life half-lived.
—the movie "Strictly Ballroom"

Houston, Summer 1987: A silver film filtered the glare of the grueling Houston sun as I stared out at a busy Richmond Avenue. Like a mirror, the reflective glass revealed my blue eyes and my six-foot, four-inch frame, tanned and fit from my years at the landscaping company, curled into an uncomfortable chair. But my eyes didn't linger on my reflection long, darting nervously around the room, as opposed to my foot tapping the floor and my hands gripping the arms of the chair.

As I sat and waited at the Montrose Clinic for the results of an HIV-AIDS test, I sensed the very walls around me thrumming with fear: the fear of all the other men and women who waited here for the news that they might be sick, that they might die. Once I understood that a virus caused AIDS I assumed I too would die of it one day. And why not: I tended bar through the wildest nights, and until recently injected speed directly into my veins.

The past ten years had disappeared in a fog of drugs, booze, and parties. My grandmother remembered me as a quiet and polite child, and I was still shy when I entered El Centro Junior College in downtown Dallas during the late 1970s. College introduced me to psychology, philosophy, and the human potential movement, and I loved what I heard. I dropped pre-med in favor of psychology. I also experimented with methamphetamines: "uppers" or "speed." Certain I had life figured out, I danced away from the chairmanship of the student council, from selection as a prominent student of the year, and a potential scholarship to Southern Methodist University, eventually dropping out entirely to deal drugs.

Drugs and alcohol reduced my shyness. For the first time I felt I "belonged," and all it took was a few hits of speed to join the "in" crowd. I failed miserably as a drug dealer, giving away more crystal meth than I sold, but I had fun, laughs, and good times.

My popularity soared when I moved to Houston and became bartender to the fabulous. Everyone knew me; I was famous (or infamous). I was also a mess. I caught hepatitis B at a cocaine "shooting party" and shared needles with friends who had since died from AIDS. Finally, in early 1987 I hit rock bottom. Unable to trust the love of friends and family, I succumbed to self-imposed isolation and became desperate with fear and loneliness. I knew I needed help or I would kill myself.

Fortunately, my friend Gary D. took me to an Alcoholics Anonymous meeting, and the hope I heard there gave me the courage to make some changes in my own life. I began life anew, clean and sober. The next step was facing the truth about my HIV status. My roommate at the time, Dr. Wayne, kept assuring me that I seemed too healthy to be HIV-positive, and so I finally surrendered to a test. Hoping against all odds to hear good news, I sat anxiously in the clinic and waited, looking out the window.

Then, a miracle. Despite all the bad choices I'd made, I am HIV-negative. Stammering my thanks to the counselor, my mind cleared as the anxiety drained from my body. Relief flooded my senses with a rush of energy. I felt ecstatic, bristling with energy. I knew I had experienced a miracle, to be healthy in the face of so much sickness and death—I'd been given a reprieve from the executioner. I walked into the Houston sunlight not noticing the scorching heat.

Many of us have had these moments of crisis, instances in which a split second determines the course of our lives: waiting for the results of a biopsy, the fracturing news of divorce, the cold certainty of death, selection for a favored job, a hair's breadth from termination. The "coulda, woulda, shouldas" crowd in to remind us of our choices. In these moments we are naked, vulnerable to absolute truth. Blessedly, not all of us have faced the executioner as I have. But life is a choice. Day in and day out we are pelted with options, some of them harsh, each with its own consequences. So I left the Montrose Clinic that day knowing that Mystery had placed her hand on me. That the gifts I'd been given in this life should no longer be squandered. The choice offered me was to LIVE, to use my knack for talking and writing and healing to make a difference in my life and my world. I have felt that fierce burning of purpose ever since.

Flash forward a few months: I was waiting impatiently at the information desk of Whole Foods Market, an organic grocery store. To pass the time I picked up a brochure for a local massage school. I read about the benefits of massage and a career in helping other people. As I stood there the *voice* from deep within me said, "You can do this." I was surprised at the voice's clarity. As a child I *knew* things before they happened. I often felt and understood things that other people didn't seem to notice. As I grew up, the more I trusted and followed my hunches, and the more I relied on them for guidance. Eventually my intuition evolved into a voice deep in my mind, encouraging me to overcome my doubts and believe in my capabilities.

Sobriety agreed with me. The dull fog I lived in for so many years lifted. My original plan was to return to college and finish my undergraduate degree in psychology, then obtain a master's in social work and start a counseling practice. Yet here I stood in the grocery store, hearing the voice and knowing my life had taken a new twist.

After checking out the local massage scene I enrolled at the Winters School. Over the next six months Nancy Winters and her friends, Joe Lindley, Debbie Starrett, Don La Guarta, Pete Lidvall, and Dr. Liang introduced me to the wonderful world of massage. For them massage was not just therapeutic touch; it was a spiritual practice. I explored the place where my body (long ignored), my mind (long indulged), my feelings (long buried), and my spirit (long denied) were interconnected. I experienced how touch called forth forgotten memories and soothed my mind, so that my body could heal and my heart could open. As my mind relaxed I began to unlock the shackles of fear that confined my life. Through massage therapy I learned how to awaken my body and call forth all the dormant energies at the center of my life, how to discipline my mind, to express and acknowledge my emotions—in brief, how to caress my spirit and let it soar.

Our yearning for the answers to questions like *"Who am I?" "What is the meaning of life?" "How can I be happy?" "What's my life purpose?"* (or as the song asks, *"What's it all about, Alfie?"*) calls us to explore and seek the heart of our relationships, to understand the mystical experience of truth. We are all taking that journey together, and occasionally our paths cross. Simply by reading this book you have signaled your willingness to stretch and reach for happiness and healing. I hope I can reinforce that resolve by encouraging you to move your body and thereby hear your own inner voice, for the best teachings in the world are useless without action.

We are often victims of our conflicting desires, and how we reconcile those desires defines the path of our happiness. For instance, I have always believed in monogamous relationships, but once I lived with a man who believed in open marriages. It was never about who was right or wrong, but what was important to me. On the one hand I wanted a life with him, but such a life went against my convictions. After much struggle I chose the way that was true for me, realizing that my deepest beliefs were more important than any of the other gifts we shared.

Fear no longer paralyzes me but instead serves as a warning signal that I have a choice.

I wrote *Body Brilliance* as a testament to love and healing: that by sharing the story of my journey to overcome fear and pain I could offer you the exercises and practices that continue to inspire and sustain me. I sincerely hope that they will give you the courage to embrace a fuller, richer, and happier life of your own.

In Service, Alan Davidson

1

BODY BRILLIANCE

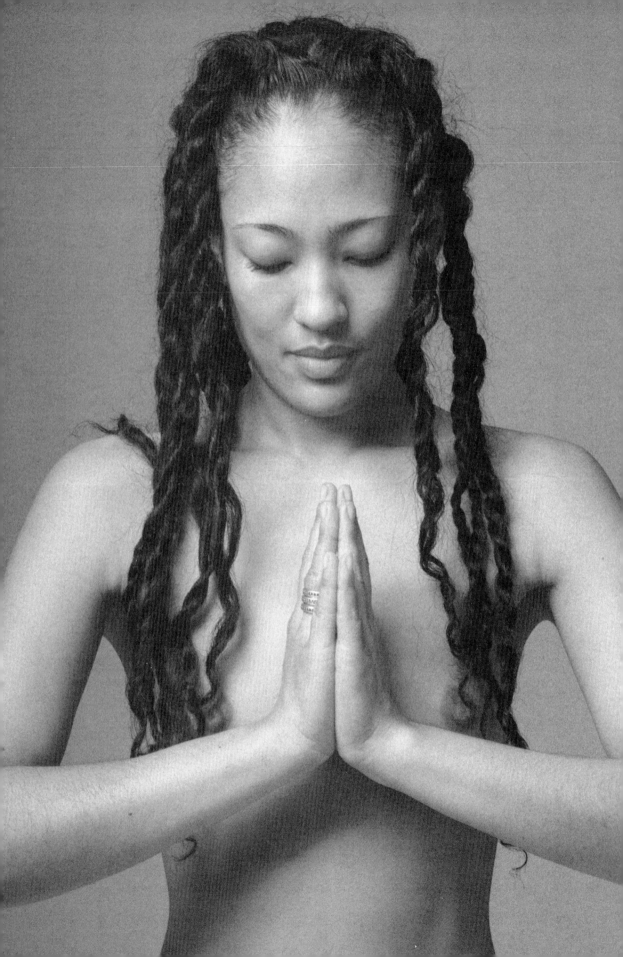

CHAPTER 1

The Five
Vital Intelligences

The strongest, surest way to the soul is through the flesh.
—Mabel Dodge, *Leonardo in Taos*

Rome, Italy: On September 7, 1960, Wilma Rudolph made Olympic history by becoming the first woman, not to mention the first African-American woman, to win three gold medals. Her accomplishments in track and field—taking first place in the 100-meter and 200-meter dash races and in the 400-meter relay—opened the door for women and girls in previously all-male track and field events. Graceful, fast and slender, the Italian press called her *La Gazzella*, the gazelle.

"Gazelle" would not have been young Wilma's nickname, however. Born in segregated Clarksville, Tennessee, on June 23, 1940, the twentieth of twenty-two children, she weighed just four-and-a-half pounds. Her parents were hardworking but quite poor. Wilma's mother nursed her sickly child through the measles, chicken pox, double pneumonia, and scarlet fever. When Wilma's left foot and leg drew up and turned in, the diagnosis of polio seemed final. Doctors gave the little girl no hope of ever walking without braces or crutches, if at all.

But her mother didn't accept the doctors' prognosis. Twice a week for two years she drove Wilma the fifty miles to Nashville for treatment at Meharry Hospital, a black medical college. The doctors showed Mrs. Rudolph how to exercise Wilma's muscles, and she in turn demonstrated the therapies to other family members.

Everyone helped, and by age eight Wilma was not only walking unaided but was also playing basketball in the backyard.

Wilma joined her junior high basketball team, but the coach didn't put her in a single game. By her sophomore year in high school Wilma started as guard. Her performance caught the attention of Ed Temple, coach of the Tennessee State University Tigerbells, who offered her a full scholarship when she graduated. Besides guiding the basketball team to a championship Wilma also excelled at track and field, earning a spot in the 1956 Olympics in Melbourne, Australia, where the sixteen-year-old brought home a bronze medal in the 400-meter relay.

But it was her outstanding accomplishments in the 1960 Olympics in Rome that brought Rudolph fame and influence. When her hometown of Clarksville wanted to have a parade in her honor, Rudolph insisted that the celebration be open to whites and blacks, not just one or the other as was customary; the parade and dinner following were the first integrated events in Clarksville. Rudolph returned to Tennessee State and earned her bachelor's degree in education in 1963. She was a lifelong advocate of racial and gender equality. Rudolph died on November 12, 1994, of brain cancer at age fifty-four.

Rudolph's successful pursuit of her athletic goals, coupled with her mother's fierce determination, serve as a testament to the body's capacity for greatness when the power of physical energy is in harmony with one's emotional and spiritual centers. Such alignment allows not only health and well-being but the knowledge that we can count on our bodies as the foundation for further development. In Wilma Rudolph's case, developing her physical capabilities probably saved her life.

These levels of energy represent the layers of our "intelligences." According to Howard Gardner in his book *Frames of Mind: The Theory of Multiple Intelligences,* humans do not have just mental intelligence—the ability for thinking and learning—but emotional, physical, and spiritual intelligences: the potential for being fit, for seeing themselves through others' eyes, for the journey toward contentment and enlightenment. I would add moral intelligence to Gardner's list: a level of intelligence that enables not only understanding of another's pain but also the desire for justice.

The Tantric philosophy of India describes five distinct koshas, or layers of consciousness, weaving together to create our human lives. The performance psychologist Jim Loehr and media guru Tony Schwartz point out the value of physical, emotional, mental, and spiritual energy in their book *The Power of Full Engagement,* joining Gardner in a contemporary explanation of what the yogis explained in their ancient texts: that each of us, although unique, is a bundle of intelligences that can be felt, measured, and fully experienced.

I've distilled these principles into *Five Vital Intelligences*. These five essential IQs—physical, emotional, mental, moral, and spiritual—represent the sum total of energized living. These layers of intelligence are nested one within the other—the physical and densest layer holding the others. Each of them is a layer of consciousness, a field of quantum energy, a capacity for growth, and an often-unrealized potential. And although few of us have succeeded in maximizing even one of our vital intelligences, much less all of them, it's never too late.

So just what are the five intelligences?

1. *The Physical.* Physical intelligence controls our body's ability to stand upright, walk, turn, twist, bend and, as in Wilma Rudolph's triumph, to run. The body's densest layer of intelligence, it is the body we see: bones, muscles, tendons, joints, and limbs—in other words, our structures, our gross anatomy.

2. *The Emotional.* Emotional intelligence principally covers the body's systemic responses, such as circulation, respiration, digestion, reproduction, and elimination. Unconscious nerve reactions like pain or pleasure fall into this category as well, as do the basic emotions of anger, sexual arousal, and the "fight or flight" response.

Actualizing emotional intelligence also encompasses what Daniel Goleman, author of *Emotional Intelligence: Why It Can Matter More Than IQ,* defines as "emotional brilliance": the development of our own emotional self coupled with the ability to empathize and redirect someone else's emotions. Rage is especially difficult to control; even trained hostage negotiators cannot say with certainty what tips an angry gunman to surrender or to self-destruct. As evidence of such skill, Richard Strozzi-Heckler, co-founder of the Lomi School, recounts this story from his friend Terry Dobson, who lived in Tokyo during the 1950s.

Dobson was one of the first Americans to learn *aikido*, an ancient Japanese martial art devoted solely to self-defense. While riding the subway one afternoon, a large, aggressive, and very drunk man got on the train. Staggering and cursing, he swung at a woman holding a baby, sending her sprawling, and frightened the remaining passengers. Dobson stood up to take on the man, believing this was definitely a case of self-defense, but stopped when the drunk decided to teach the "foreigner some Japanese manners." The drunk was about to slug Dobson when someone yelled "Hey!" in a cheery voice.

Spinning around to see who called him, the drunk found a small man in a kimono, probably in his seventies, smiling at him. He waved the drunk to come sit with him, asking what the man had been drinking. The drunk rudely answered, "Sake, and it's none of your business," but the old gentleman didn't let on and began extolling the virtues of sake and how he and his wife enjoyed opening a bottle in their garden. He rambled on about his garden and the persimmon tree there until the drunk's anger began to recede. The drunk admitted that he, too, liked persimmons, and when the old man commented that his new companion's wife was probably lovely as well, the man revealed that his wife had died.

When Dobson left the subway, the formerly violent drunk had his head in the old gentleman's lap, sobbing about his late wife, his lost job, and his overwhelming shame. Using no force or even harsh words, the old Japanese gentleman had completely diffused the situation by simply being there for the other man, giving the drunk his sympathy and undivided attention. Such skill exemplifies human connection and true emotional brilliance.

3. *The Mental.* Mental intelligence refers, plainly enough, to the thinking mind or cognition, but also includes the functions of the subconscious mind and the inspirations of the super-conscious mind. This third vital intelligence encompasses the nerves and the brain, whose mysterious, amazing functions facilitate communication, memory, and information retrieval. Mental consciousness also includes the search for knowledge and the development of one's education.

Considered the greatest thinker and scientist of the twentieth century, and maybe for all time, Albert Einstein represented the development of a highly refined mental intelligence tempered by his modest, unassuming personality and spiritual humility. For Einstein, scientific endeavor only heightened what he called true art: the search for the mysterious.

Einstein (1879–1955) was born in the German city of Ulm. His parents, Hermann and Pauline, were non-observant Jews that placed their son in a Catholic elementary school. Young Albert was often tagged a slow learner, but rumors of his failure at math are untrue. At age five, Hermann gave his son a compass, and Einstein credited his fascination with the unseen "something" that controlled the needle as one of the revelatory experiences of his life. He dropped out of school before graduation, at odds with the European educational practice of rote memorization. Einstein later re-enrolled in school in Switzerland, finishing a year later.

In 1896, Einstein entered the University of Zurich, where he met a young Serbian woman named Mileva Maric, the only woman at the university that year to pursue the same program as Einstein. He described her as his equal. They became lovers and had a daughter, Lieserl, in January 1902. Einstein relinquished his German citizenship in 1896 and became a Swiss citizen in 1901. Albert and Mileva married in 1903; Mileva bore two sons—Hans Albert (1904) and Eduard (1910). Unable to find a teaching post after graduation, Einstein became an assistant technical examiner at the Swiss Patent Office.

Einstein described 1905 as his "miracle year," publishing four articles that became the foundation of modern physics. The first, on the photoelectric effect, proved the existence of photons and confirmed scientist Max Planck's theory of quantum energy. The second explored Brownian motion and provided empirical proof of the existence of atoms, converting even the most ardent "anti-atomists."

The third paper, "On the Electrodynamics of Moving Bodies," introduced the world to Einstein's theory of relativity. Einstein's lectures at the Prussian Academy of Sciences in 1915 on relativity theory concluded with his replacement of Newton's law of gravity: no longer was gravity a force but a function of the curvature of space and time. The British scientist Arthur Eddington confirmed Einstein's theory in 1919 when Eddington measured how much the light emanating from a star was bent by the sun's gravity when it passed close to the sun, an effect called gravitational lensing. When the *New York Times* published the results of Eddington's experiments, Einstein's fame was assured.

The fourth paper, "Does the Inertia of a Body Depend Upon its Energy Content?," outlined Einstein's famous equation: $E = mc^2$, or the energy of a body at rest equals its mass times the square of the speed of light. Any of these papers could have earned Einstein a Nobel Prize in physics, but the committee recognized Einstein with a Nobel in 1921 specifically for his work on the photoelectric effect—no doubt because Einstein's other theories were as yet too controversial.

Einstein divorced Mileva in 1919 and married his first cousin Elsa. He returned to teach in Berlin, reclaiming his German citizenship, but fled the Nazis and emigrated to America in 1933. Einstein taught at Princeton University until his death, becoming an American citizen in 1940 (he kept his Swiss citizenship, however), where he continued to publish papers and push the envelope of accepted physical theory.

Those who knew Einstein described him as kind, friendly, and modest. His wild, white hair, moth-eaten sweaters, and ability to concentrate solely on his thoughts are iconic with the absent-minded professor. Politically Einstein was a social democrat, believing in a world economy and government with emphasis on human rights. Although he petitioned President Franklin Roosevelt to consider the development of an atomic bomb before the Nazis did, he embraced pacifism and opposed nuclear testing and armament.

Einstein supported Zionism and other Jewish causes and was invited to be the second president of the new state of Israel: the only American offered a position as a foreign head of state. Nevertheless, he did not observe the religiosities of Judaism but instead believed in a great mysterious spirituality that he felt should surround all men, particularly those who sought scientific proof.

In an essay reprinted in 1931, Einstein mused:

> *A knowledge of the existence of something we cannot penetrate, our perceptions of the profoundest reason and the most radiant beauty, which only in their most primitive forms are accessible to our minds—it is this knowledge and this emotion that constitute true religiosity; in this sense alone, I am a deeply religious man.*

Although we remember Einstein for his astounding theories and proofs, he did not let his mental intelligence eclipse his sense of wonder about the depth of man's incapacity to know everything. His ability to concentrate prevented his conscious mind from succumbing to irrelevant chatter and foolish opinion. Most of us may never achieve Einstein's brilliance, but we can refine our cognitive abilities and turn our sharpened talents to better understanding the mysteries of ourselves and of the universe.

4. *The Moral.* The fourth vital intelligence represents discernment, our ability to distinguish right from wrong and make the correct choice based on more than just facts. This level of intelligence reflects our values, our behaviors, our purpose in life, and how we recognize the rights and worth of others. Moral intelligence is characterized by the growth from selfish concern for "me" to interest in others and ultimately caring for everyone. The "little voice" of our conscience speaks from this intelligence as well.

Sometimes that voice calls out so loudly that one cannot stifle it with the noise of the status quo. For Mel White, an evangelical Christian pastor, seminary professor, author, and ghostwriter for prominent evangelists like Jerry Falwell, Billy Graham, Oliver North, and Pat Robertson, his conscience kept telling him that hiding his homosexuality in the fundamentalist closet was wrong.

So when White was challenged to speak out against Christian fundamentalist ideas about gays; to live openly as a gay man in front of his former evangelical friends and co-workers; to speak to hostile audiences; to fast or protest on the steps of the Capitol or at the gates of the White House—he accepted the mission.

In 2002, White and his partner of 20 years, Gary Nixon, leased a house across the street from Jerry Falwell's church, Thomas Street Baptist, in Lynchburg, Virginia. Every Sunday White and Nixon brought gay and lesbian worshippers to services so that members of the congregation met them on a person-to-person basis.

Falwell didn't like it (he and White are not close friends anymore), but White's efforts are slowly bearing fruit. The movement, called Soulforce and boasting chapters in over twenty communities, draws on the principles of love and civil disobedience put forth by Mahatma Mohandas Gandhi and executed by Martin Luther King Jr. White sees his goal as acceptance for the gay/lesbian/bisexual/transgender community, as well as permission for its members to seek justice for themselves. As Mark Twain once remarked, "Of going along to get along, maintaining silence that obscures the truth ... is timid—and shabby."

Mel White probably doesn't consider himself a hero, but sacrificing his comfortable position for what he knew was right took radical courage. His honesty reminds us that recognizing one's moral intelligence is a vital guidepost on the path to development of body and soul.

5. *The Spiritual.* This fifth intelligence embraces the mysterious life force, the subtle knowledge of the divine and man's relation to that wisdom. In the Hindu chakra system this life energy is called *prana;* to the Chinese it is *chi,* and for Westerners it is the *auric field:* all descriptions of the magical, spiritual connection between humans and something greater than themselves.

A shining example of spiritual brilliance is the thirteenth century Sufi Jalaluddin Rumi, still revered today as a man completely attuned to the subtleties of the spirit and the joyous recognition of those connections with one another.

Rumi was born into a distinguished family on September 30, 1207, in Balkh, now part of Afghanistan. Torn by the chaos of the Christian Crusades, threats to the Ottoman Empire and the usual doses of graft and corruption, the early thirteenth century was a period of great turmoil. Fleeing the Mongol armies of Genghis Khan when young Rumi was twelve, he and his family wandered for ten years over Persia, Arabia, and Asia Minor.

The boy learned the ways of a Sufi, living with a master until he had learned what each teacher could impart and then traveled on to the next. By the year 1244 Rumi had succeeded his esteemed father as a great scholar and head of a college. He excelled in mathematics, physics, law, astronomy, Arabic and Persian language and grammar, Koranic studies, jurisprudence, music, and poetry. His knowledge of Sufi ways gave him leadership over many disciples. And he could have spent the rest of his life secure in his position and the fame and adulation it generated.

But that was not to be. In December 1244, Rumi met Shams-i-Tabriz, a wandering dervish and spiritual explorer—the "ultimate theological hippie," according to Jean Huston in her book *The Search for the Beloved*. Rumi recognized in Shams the total sublimation of self into the spirit of the divine, and he fell instantly in love. Rumi described this love as being burned, cooked, annihilated, yet he was ecstatic to have found one who so completely and intensely transformed him.

Shams, which means "sun," was an itinerant mystic in his sixties when he met Rumi, a well-respected young scholar and head of the college in Konya, now part of Turkey. In *The Way of Passion,* author and Rumi scholar Andrew Harvey speculated that Shams had been totally enlightened and needed a disciple, a mouthpiece capable of receiving the burning immensity of his knowledge. Shams may have begged God to give him this man, this crucible for his fire, and offered his life to God in return.

Although several accounts of their meeting exist, Harvey preferred the one that had Rumi riding a donkey on his way to the bazaar, accompanied by his students on foot. Shams ran after him and, grabbing the bridle, quizzed the teacher with a riddle, asking quite madly whether Rumi thought Mohammed or the Sufi mystic Bayazid was the greater. Rumi answered conventionally that Mohammed was the Prophet, therefore the greater. But Shams demanded, "What is the meaning then of this?" The prophet said to God, "I have not known thee as I should have," and Bayazid said, "Glory be to me. How high is my dignity." Rumi remembered that Mohammed had regretted not knowing the Sufi better—in other words, that the prophet revered Bayazid, making the Sufi the more enlightened of the two.

At this, Rumi supposedly fainted and fell off the donkey; when he regained consciousness, he took Shams' hand and walked with him to a private cell at the college, where the two men communed in ecstatic harmony for forty days—Shams transmitting his knowledge of the divine with the intensity, violence, and speed required of a man who knew he would die soon, and Rumi received all of that wisdom in his open heart.

Jealousy and hatred overcame Rumi's disciples, however, prompting Shams to leave abruptly. Rumi went insane with grief, seeking his beloved everywhere. After months of searching, he learned Shams was in Damascus, and he sent his second son, Sultan Walad, to bring him back. Their reunion was as joyous as the first meeting, and they sang and danced and shared the divine mysteries. Again the disciples' jealousy outran their love for Rumi, and in December 1247 they probably murdered the mystic. He was never seen again.

Rumi once more descended into madness, weeping and whirling to cope with his grief. The whirling, attributed to Rumi and practiced by Sufi dervishes thereafter, was thought to bring space and time into the center of God's being. Rumi also wrote some of the world's most beautiful poetry in an effort to heal his pain. Eventually, however, Rumi understood that Shams had imparted all he had, and that Rumi, cleansed in the fire of his agony and loss, had been redeemed in the light of divine love.

Rumi wrote:

Love is an infinite Sea whose skies are a bubble of foam.
...Without Love, nothing in the world
would have life.
...Every single atom is drunk on this
Perfection and runs toward It
And what does this running secretly say
but "Glory be to God."

Every one of us, in our heart of hearts, may suffer the excruciating pain of abandonment—the searing separation from God—that comes from our often feeble attempts at enlightenment. The redemption of Jalaluddin Rumi reminds us that peaking our spiritual intelligence soothes our fears and helps bridge the chasm of separation. Such is the goal of every seeker of truth.

But can actualization of these five layers of vital intelligence—through our bodies—really create a union of flesh and spirit? Scientists agree that *life is energy.* And no matter whether one chooses to develop one or all of the body's intelligences, the central premise is that these energies come from and are developed *through the body.* It's our factory, our temple, our repository of whatever we do, good or bad. We know each of these intelligences by their noticeable quality of energy: we can feel physically charged, emotionally thrilled, mentally crisp, morally engaged, and spiritually vital.

Our energy at each level of intelligence is our marker and our measure of how we are fulfilling the potential of that layer. Are we living into the full promise of that intelligence, or are we running on fumes in that area of our lives?

Imagine a ceiling fan, the five separate blades circulating around the hub. As they turn, however, the five whirling blades blur into a single image. The center of the fan is unaffected by the spinning blades, much like the stillness of God's being in the center of the dervish's whirling body. Nevertheless, the fan blades—while connected to the center—are separate, each wobbling a bit differently from the other four.

Similarly, the five vital intelligences each have their own vibrations or frequencies, and each possesses its own techniques for success. But taken together, these five levels create an eternal, constant center: what Asian mystics and quantum physicists call "the pure stillness of being" or the "stillness within all movement." Such a core is the beginning and the end, the doorway to the pure energy of life and the total of our lives' efforts, the yin and yang, the alpha and omega: the level of enlightenment that Shams knew and the rest of us hope to realize.

But then that is the purpose of the *Body Brilliance* series (you're reading volume 1): to demonstrate exercises and techniques designed to work through our bodies—for that is where the five intelligences lie—in order to heal and actualize these five layers of consciousness into a harmonic whole. Overcoming the inertia of daily living takes a tremendous amount of energy. But when that energy is redirected and aligned, our own wobbly vibrations blend into one shining pursuit: the happiness gained from living an extraordinary life.

The exercises and examples presented throughout the *Body Brilliance* series serve as a means to shine the importance of these five layers of intelligence to living a wonderful life. Each one is vital to the support and development of the others, but that doesn't mean any one of these actualizations would not be a worthy goal on its own. Elevating the five intelligences seems deceptively simple, but knowledge alone is insufficient. Reaching a peak experience requires work, dedication, and desire. *Body Brilliance* is the art and science of growing each of these intelligences to our highest abilities and harmonizing them together. Following the routines in this series, however, helps your efforts immensely. And the results are a radiant life—happy, healthy, and ultimately gratifying.

Visit www.BodyBrillianceBook.com to read about other masters of body brilliance. Better yet: post stories telling about your own inspirations.

FURTHER READING

"Albert Einstein." Wikipedia, the free encyclopedia. Available online at http://wikipedia.org/wiki/Albert_Einstein.

Gardner, Howard. *Frames of Mind: The Theory of Multiple Intelligences.* New York: BasicBooks, 1983.

Goleman, Daniel. *Emotional Intelligence: Why It Can Matter More Than IQ.* New York: Bantam Books, 1995.

Harvey, Andrew. *The Way of Passion: A Celebration of Rumi.* Berkeley, CA: Frog Ltd. Publishing, 1994.

Huston, Jean. *The Search for the Beloved: Journeys in Mythology and Sacred Psychology.* Los Angeles: Jeremy P. Tarcher Inc., 1987.

Loehr, Jim, and Tony Schwartz. *The Power of Full Engagement: Managing Energy, Not Time, Is the Key to High Performance and Personal Renewal.* New York: Simon & Schuster, 2003.

"Wilma Rudolph." Available online at http://www.africanamericans.com/Profiles.html.

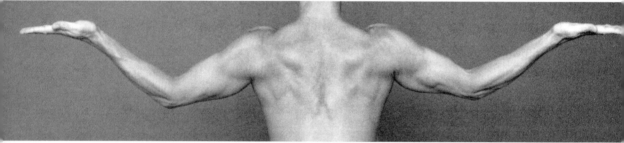

CHAPTER 2

Happiness
Is...

The Constitution only guarantees the American people the right to
pursue happiness. You have to catch it yourself.
—Benjamin Franklin

We humans prize happiness more than anything else. We seek it for its own sake, and we pursue all our other goals—romance, power, money, and health—because we believe they will make us happy. The Greek philosopher Aristotle agreed with this opinion over 2,300 years ago, and little seems to have changed since the first toga party.

But what is happiness, this glittering prize we humans so long for? We often take it for granted as an end in itself, but happiness can be difficult to explain, hard to achieve and perhaps impossible to hold onto. For me, happiness is a state of being: enjoyment of everything life offers. It allows for making the most of life's difficulties and celebrating life's pleasures. Although defining happiness could require an entire dictionary, we can understand happiness through the body's vital intelligences: as a sensual pleasure, a feeling, an attitude, a behavior, and a vibration.

Happiness at the physical layer of intelligence simply means the enjoyment of our bodily pleasures. Imagine these sensations: touching silk fabric, tasting a crisp apple, smelling a spring bouquet of flowers, dancing at a party, or listening to a favorite piece of music. Just listing these activities triggers positive emotions. Satisfying our bodily pleasures is the source of an immediate, delicious, sensual happiness, but alas, such responses are fleeting and cannot deliver long-lasting contentment. Martin

Seligman, in *Authentic Happiness,* says, "Neurons are wired to respond to novel events." The neurons—and the brain itself at this layer of intelligence—seek a constant stream of new and varied pleasures.

At intelligence level two, the emotional layer, we experience happiness as well being, contentment, and joy: the positive feelings that make life enjoyable. But to know happiness only as an emotion means that our delight is temporary, rising and falling with our moods.

After returning to college to finish my bachelor's degree, I spent some time in Guilin, China, working on a senior project. Though I love travel and exotic adventures, three weeks of Chinese sights, smells, and foods left me longing for home. One night after returning to Hong Kong I spied the Golden Arches down a busy street. My pace quickened as I thrilled at the thought: "A hamburger, an American hamburger." In Hong Kong, late at night, good old American junk food was the best I was going to get. Fortunately, the menu was spelled out in pictures and both English and Chinese words. I ordered a hamburger, french fries, and a chocolate shake.

As I waited for my fast food (though it couldn't come fast enough), I remembered eating in our dormitory in Guilin. Our professor at the university, Dr. Wright, was highly esteemed, and as his students we were held in great respect. Our hosts considered us honored guests, and we ate better fare than the Chinese students. There were the constant rounds of rice noodles, soups, different meats, and unfamiliar sauces. Often these foods were quite tasty but nevertheless remained a mystery. The webbing of duck's feet, a delicacy in Guilin, was delicious, but I'm just glad I didn't know what I was eating until I had finished. (I did manage to avoid the "grilled poisonous snake" in the open street markets.)

Finally, my tray arrived, and I savored the moment. I hadn't eaten in a McDonald's in a decade, since I rarely ate beef or fried foods. The burger came with ketchup, and my first bite was heaven. The entire meal was scrumptious. It's not that the food was even that tasty, or that I was really that hungry. Or even that I wanted to experience just the physical pleasure of eating. It was the return to home, to civilization as I knew it, garish and cheap as only a McDonald's could be. I loved it. I felt warmly happy and satisfied. But my passing feeling of happiness, sitting in that McDonald's in Hong Kong, represented merely emotional satisfaction. As fabulous as it was, it was fleeting. It just didn't last.

Experiencing happiness through the third or mental intelligence requires us to consciously choose joy: to focus on the positive aspects of our lives, or as the old song says, to "accentuate the positive" and "eliminate the negative." The following bit of wisdom, which has probably made the rounds of every mailbox on the Internet, exemplifies this choice:

She is ninety-two years old, petite, well poised, and proud. She is fully dressed each morning by eight o'clock, with her hair fashionably coiffed and her makeup perfectly applied, despite the fact that she is legally blind.

Today she has moved to a nursing home. Her husband of seventy years recently passed away, making this move necessary. After many hours of waiting patiently in the lobby of the nursing home, where I am employed, she smiled sweetly when told her room was ready. As she maneuvered her walker to the elevator, I provided a visual description of her tiny room, including the eyelet curtains that had been hung on her window. "I love it," she stated with the enthusiasm of an eight-year-old having just been presented with a new puppy.

"Mrs. Jones, you haven't seen the room yet; just wait," I said. Then she spoke these words that I will never forget. "That does not have anything to do with it," she gently replied. "Happiness is something you decide on ahead of time. Whether I like my room or not does not depend on how the furniture is arranged. It is how I arrange my mind. I have already decided to love it.

"It is a decision I make every morning when I wake up. I have a choice. I can spend the day in bed recounting the difficulty I have with the parts of my body that no longer work, or I can get out of bed and be thankful for the ones that do work. Each day is a gift, and as long as my eyes open, I will focus on the new day and all of the happy memories I have stored away just for this time in my life. Old age is like a bank account. You withdraw from it what you have already put in."

We realize happiness in the moral layer of intelligence by performing a thousand acts of kindness. Aristotle, seeking the answer to the question "What is the good life for man," studied the behavior and conversations of average people in their everyday lives. On the basis of what he saw, the great philosopher defined happiness as "an activity of the soul in accord with perfect virtue." Aristotle understood that committing ourselves to our best virtues, as we understand them, every day, gives us a happy life.

But happiness in and of itself is not the destination; it is the by-product of our actions and intentions. The Austrian psychologist Viktor Frankl, in his book *Man's Search for Meaning,* compares happiness to success, recommending, "Don't aim at success—the more you aim at it and make it a target, the more you are going to miss it. For success, like happiness, cannot be pursued; it must ensue … as the unintended side effect of one's personal dedication to a course greater than oneself."

I enjoy helping people. Once I loaned a friend $1,000 for his tuition to massage school. He quickly defaulted on the loan. After a year or so of badgering him to repay the loan, and worse, suffering the gnawing anger and resentment I felt toward him, I had had enough. I wrote him a letter absolving him of his debt and asked that when the time came to repay the money, that he give it to a charity of his choosing. Releasing those emotions gave me surprising relief.

In the old TV show "Kung Fu," Master Po instructs his young pupil Caine to take on the "obligation of ten." For an act of kindness done to him, Caine was obliged to return, over time, ten other acts of kindness. I have turned the relief I felt from absolving that unpaid debt into other good turns. Now when I help someone out in some way, rather than ask for repayment in kind, I invite them to "pay it forward": to help someone else in the future. I trust the gift will ripple out into the world.

This quote from Dean Koontz's book *From the Corner of His Eye* speaks to the power of kindness:

> *Each smallest act of kindness reverberates across great distances and spans of time, affecting lives unknown to the one whose generous spirit was the source of this good echo, because kindness is passed on and grows each time it's passed, until a simple courtesy becomes an act of selfless courage years later and far away.*

It's no wonder these small kindnesses, given often and regularly, add tremendously to my happiness.

Happiness expressed through our spiritual intelligence is best understood vibrationally. David R. Hawkins, M.D., Ph.D., developed a vibrational "map of consciousness," which he outlined in his revolutionary book *Power vs. Force: The Hidden Determinants of Human Behavior.* Hawkins calibrated the range of possible human vibrations, or spiritual intelligence, on a scale from one to 1,000: a vibration of one is very near death; a vibration of 1,000 was the highest possible frequency of consciousness for mankind. Each vibrational range had a corresponding emotional level. Through Hawkins's work we can actually measure the growth of spiritual intelligence. Here is a brief sketch of the "map":

Emotional Level	Vibrational Log
Enlightenment	700 to 1000
Peace	600
Joy	540
Love	500
Reason	400
Courage	200
Pride	175
Anger	150
Fear	100
Grief	75
Guilt	30
Shame	20

Spiritual intelligence vibrating below 200, the level of courage, was "life depleting" and considered negative. Consciousness vibrating above 200 was "life affirming" and considered positive. The vibration level of 200 was the tipping point in attuning our awareness. Vibrationally speaking, happiness occurred when our conscious state of being peaked between frequencies of 500 to 540, or between love and joy. In Japanese, the word *sartori* represented a temporary experience of enlightenment, spiking into the 700-plus range of vibration.

Each vibration was also logarithmic. Hawkins wrote, "The calibration figures do not represent an arithmetic but a logarithmic progression. Thus, a level of 300 is not twice the amplitude of 150; it is 300 to the tenth power (300^{10})." Raising the vibration a few degrees meant a substantial increase in power.

Dr. Hawkins's "map of consciousness" is just one yardstick to measure our journey of spiritual evolution. We may be fortunate enough to experience the states of higher vibration: love, extended happiness, even sartori. But these experiences, often all too brief, are signposts to show us the way. They give us a taste and feel of "the high life," of an enlightened life that fulfills its potential.

The rush of the high explains why drugs are so popular. They produce a temporary euphoria, which are usually followed by some crashing low. Afterwards we return to the reality of our lives; there is rarely an evolutionary shift in vibration. Sadly, the hope that drugs might be the path to happiness often leads to disaster—and the loss of happiness.

I'd studied spiritual principles for ten years, had been in therapy for more than that, and yet I was not happy. But when I gave up trying to transcend my body, when I gave up denying the reality of my body and its pleasures, when I shifted my focus to live in and through my body, I began to see real changes in my health and happiness. Once my focus shifted, my behaviors changed. And so did my life.

Spiritual contentment and evolution are like happiness and success. They are ephemeral and cannot be grasped. The more we strive for them, the further they slide out of reach. It is when we focus our attention, engage our hearts, and commit our lives to the "something greater than ourselves" that our vibrational frequencies rise, steadily and consistently. We eventually live into the states of love, happiness, peace, and the bliss of unity.

FURTHER READING

Aristotle. *Ethics*. Bath, England: The Folio Society, 2003.

Csikszentmihalyi, Mihaly. *Flow: The Psychology of Optimal Experience*. New York: Harper & Row, 1990.

Frankl, Victor. *Man's Search for Meaning*. New York: Pocket Books, 1999.

Hawkins, David, M.D., Ph.D., *Power vs. Force: The Hidden Determinants of Human Behavior*. Sedona, AZ: Veritas, 1995.

Koontz, Dean. *From the Corner of His Eye*. New York: Bantam Books, 2001.

Seligman, Martin. *Authentic Happiness*. New York: Free Press, 2002.

We choose our joys and sorrows long before we experience them.

—Kahlil Gibran

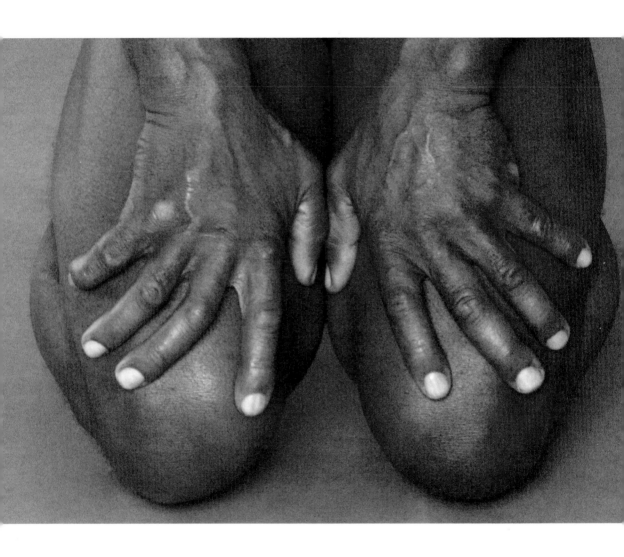

CHAPTER 3

Harmony Is Health

Health is natural, thus effortless, to the individual who
has achieved harmony between body and mind.
—Ron Perfetti

The words "health," "whole" and "holy" all share the same ancestry. *Webster's New Collegiate Dictionary* defines health as the "condition of being sound in body, mind, or spirit." We understand it more often as the absence of disease and freedom from pharmaceutical drugs. But great health is a state of extraordinary well-being. It relies on more than good nutrition and physical fitness. As George Leonard says in his essay "Towards a Balanced Way," good health involves "a vibrant flow of 'energy' throughout the body. It implies body/mind/spirit harmony."

Health and well-being are the vibrant stream of life through the subtle and gross layers of the human body: truth itself flowing optimally through each of the five vital intelligences. Each layer, in turn, is in balance and in harmony with the others. Health is effortless. It is natural law—the simple flow of energy, undiluted and unimpeded. Some limits to health are found in genetic shortcomings. But most illness and physical ailments are rooted in the blocks found within the layers of intelligence. These obstacles constrict the natural flow of energy, affecting the overall health and well-being of the body. Richard Strozzi-Heckler, co-founder of the Lomi School, sees ill health in this way:

All disease, whether physical, emotional, mental, acute, or chronic, is the result of an obstructed energy flow. The effectiveness of any healing art, therapy, or system of learning is determined by its ability to reconstitute life flow in a balanced harmonious fashion. Creativity is movement; disease is blocked movement. Healing reconnects awareness to areas lacking vitality and movement.

In Chapter Two, I introduced Dr. David Hawkins's "map of consciousness," his groundbreaking study measuring the energy frequencies, or vibrations, emitted by each of the body's emotions and spiritual intelligences. On a scale of one to 1,000—with one being near death and 1,000 being in a state of total enlightenment—happiness occurrs at frequencies of 500 to 540.

Every layer of vital intelligence emits an energetic frequency, depending on the layer's vitality, but these frequencies fluctuate with the ups and downs of day-to-day living. The specific frequencies of each layer combine to give a person his or her predominant vibration overall. Using *Body Brilliance,* one may refine and increase the frequencies of each of the body's layers of vital intelligence, creating new harmonies and raising the level of the predominant vibration.

Throughout this book I present different exercises and techniques to strengthen each layer of vital intelligence and increase that level's vibrational frequency. Weight training and yoga are just two examples of bodywork that promote fitness of the muscles, bones, and joints as well as elevating the vibrational frequency of the physical intelligence. Adopting a particular diet, learning breathing techniques, or becoming more emotionally mature facilitate development of emotional intelligence.

Our mental/cognitive intelligence could benefit from daily meditation or simply a more positive outlook. Regular acts of kindness—without expectation of formal recognition—lead to improvement in the fourth layer, or moral intelligence. And once we have learned how to increase the frequencies of the first through fourth vital intelligences, there are many esoteric exercises for raising the fifth, or spiritual, level.

Harmonizing the levels of vital intelligence, however, provides the greatest increase in the body's predominant vibration. While any individual may excel at one intelligence level over the others, such dominance will not succeed if it is gained at the expense of the other four intelligences.

Consider this: I know many bodybuilders who are muscularly well built and look great. The time and effort they take to bulk up increases the energetic frequency of the first layer of consciousness: their bones and muscles. But some of those guys smoke cigarettes or use steroids. The smoking damages lung function, and the metabolic steroids (known as "juice") interfere with the natural flow of the body's hormonal system. Either one of these habits lowers, not raises, the energetic frequency of the second layer of intelligence, and the resulting disharmony reduces a person's predominant vibration.

Here's another example of disharmony and how it can affect vibration:

During the rise of fascism in the 1930s, the Germans placed a remarkable emphasis on physical fitness. Health became a national obsession, as National Socialist (Nazi) sport clubs encouraged "true" Germans to participate in all manner of outdoor activities and exercises. Jewish athletes or other "inferiors" were forbidden to compete.

The Germans' first and second layers of intelligence thrived on such a fitness regimen, and Adolf Hitler planned to show off his "superior" Aryan athletes at the 1936 Olympics, which were held conveniently in the German capital city of Berlin. Hitler's triumph collapsed, however, when Jesse Owens, an African American sprinter, won an unprecedented four gold medals in the 100-meter dash, the 200-meter dash, the long jump, and the 400-meter relay.

Unfortunately for the German facists, their belief that they were superior to all other races lowered the frequency of the third vital intelligence: the layer of attitude and thinking. And the hatred fomented by the Nazis, as well as the commission of unspeakable crimes and the genocide of millions of Jews, gypsies, homosexuals, Communists—anyone deemed a threat to Aryan racial purity—drastically lowered the vibrational frequency of the Germans' moral intelligence. Leni Riefenstahl's documentary on Hitler, *Triumph of the Will,* became a portrait of the subjugation of the will. The disharmony and crash of the vibrations in the third and fourth layers overrode any benefits gained by Germany's physical fitness campaign.

The power of harmony—of all the layers pulsing in concert—is phenomenal. In contrast to the Nazi fiasco, Wilma Rudolph's Olympic triumph (profiled in Chapter One) not only spotlighted her physical brilliance but gave her an opportunity to work for her causes: women's sports, civil rights, women's rights, and equal opportunities. Her amazing physical accomplishments shone even more brightly when complemented by her emotional, mental, and moral excellence.

The sum of the five vital intelligences is so much greater than the highest achievement of any one of them alone. And the *Body Brilliance* series can help you develop those intelligences so that your spirit, too, will shine with health, happiness, and harmony.

Further Reading

Berenbaum, Michael. *The World Must Know: The History of the Holocaust as Told in United States Holocaust Memorial Museum.* Boston: Little, Brown and Co., 1993.

Leonard, George. "Towards a Balanced Way." *The Lomi Papers.* Mill Valley, CA: The Lomi School, 1979.

He who lives in harmony with himself lives in harmony with the universe.

—Marcus Aurelius

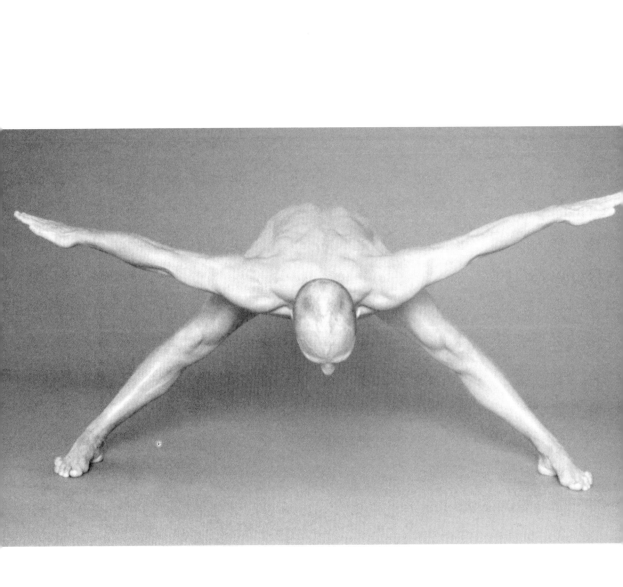

CHAPTER 4

Peaking Your Intelligences

Your capacities are trembling to be born.
—Abraham Maslow

One may measure the growth of the body and mind by many yardsticks, and each of the various spiritual and psychological development models is useful in its own way. The Hindu system of chakras defined seven levels of consciousness, associating different parts of the body with those spiritual centers (chakra means *wheel of spinning light*). The names of the chakras and their locations are:

- chakra 1 *(muladhara)*, at the base of the spine
- chakra 2 *(svadisthana)*, a few inches farther up the spine
- chakra 3 *(manipura)*, at the level of the navel
- chakra 4 *(anahata)*, at the level of the heart
- chakra 5 *(vishuddha)*, in the throat area
- chakra 6 *(ajna)*, between the eyebrows
- chakra 7 *(sahasrara*, at the top of the head.

The seven distinct levels of the chakra system can also provide a yardstick of a person's (or society's) conscious development.

- chakra 1, instinctual and tribal impulses

- chakra 2, maternal and intimate impulses

- chakra 3, the impulse to wield power (for good or bad)

- chakra 4, the impulse to care for the world

- chakra 5, the impulse to speak and live personal truth

- chakra 6, the impulse for spiritual truth

- chakra 7, the impulse for universal, mystical freedom.

The anthropologist Jean Gebser, on the other hand, narrowed spiritual development into five stages: archaic, magic, mythic, rational, and integral.

Psychologist Abraham Maslow agreed with Gebser on the number of levels —five—but he believed the concept of self-actualization depended on a different "hierarchy of needs": physiological satisfaction, security, love and a sense of belonging, self-esteem, and self-actualization. Any one of these analyses provides guidance for the growth of our vital intelligences; it all depends on how you gauge your progress.

Here's a simple example using the hierarchy of needs: as I write this, my partner, Jim, and I are about to become grandparents. Jim's only daughter will give birth to a baby girl around July Fourth. (If I have my way, she'll be the best-dressed baby girl in Baton Rouge.) But regardless of her wardrobe, we recognize that:

- As an infant, our granddaughter's basic physical needs of food, sleep, warmth, and touch must be provided first.

- The satisfaction of those basic needs allows the baby to sense the stability and order of her life, and, as she becomes a toddler, to feel secure in her position and ready to test her limits.

- With our granddaughter's basic physical and safety needs continually met, she'll reach the third stage of healthy growth: love and belonging. A child by now, she will start to look beyond her parents to her extended family and to her friends around the neighborhood and at school for affirmation of her "self."

- Once she thrives at this third stage of growth she will be ready for the fourth stage: the development of her self-esteem through self-respect and recognition by her peers. By this time our granddaughter will be a young lady (and definitely choosing her own clothes).

- Finally, our granddaughter—surrounded by love and support and possessed with a positive sense of self, all her previous needs met—will be ready to satisfy her need for "self-actualization," wherein she can confidently develop her innate talents and discover that joining with others enriches her own potential.

What is consistent in each of these models, in addition to mapping progress through the stages of growth, is the idea that once a level of development is achieved, it must remain achieved to ensure the success of each new rung climbed on the development ladder. Our higher growth rests squarely upon the solid foundation of lower-level accomplishment.

In his article "Introduction to Integral Theory and Practice," author Ken Wilber notes that:

> ... by "stages" we mean progressive and permanent milestones along the evolutionary path of your unfolding. Whether we talk stages of consciousness, stages of energy, stages of culture, stages of spiritual realization, stages of moral development, and so on, we are talking of these important and fundamental rungs in the unfolding of your higher, deeper, wider potentials.

Throughout this discussion of the body's vital intelligences it may have occurred to you how unevenly developed you are. You're really good in some layers and lacking in others. That's true for virtually all of us. Some people are excellent thinkers but may have mean, selfish personalities—not exactly beacons of morality. Some people are talented athletes but have difficulty with simple arithmetic. And some people become so enchanted with the search for their own enlightenment that they ignore the needs of their fellow travelers.

Most of us excel in one or two layers of intelligence. These are our strengths. Part of developing body brilliance involves a realistic assessment of your best talents so that you can build on that foundation. But don't overlook the areas that suffer from neglect or intentional (God forbid, pathological) wrongheadedness.

Perhaps one of the world's greatest scientific minds belonged to Sir Isaac Newton (1642–1727). Young Isaac was expected to continue the management of his father's farm, but Isaac had bigger dreams. He worked his way through Trinity College, Cambridge University, keeping a notebook of his observations and experiments in subjects barely covered by his professors. He taught himself trigonometry to better understand astrology (then a legitimate science) and studied chemistry and alchemy.

But like many other geniuses, Newton's brilliant analytical mind was often over-shadowed by his anger, insecurity, pride, obsessiveness, and vengeful nature. The infant Isaac wasn't expected to even live, much less become famous. He was born in Woolsthorpe, Lincolnshire, to Hannah Ayscough Newton; his father, Isaac Sr., died three months before his birth. Within two years the young widow had married a well-to-do minister named Barnabas Smith and moved away to start a new family. His grandmother raised young Isaac until Smith died in 1653, when his mother returned and tried to resume relations with her son, which failed miserably. Isaac hated his mother and stepfather, and later biographers attributed his psychotic behaviors to his early abandonment.

By 1671 Newton had invented a reflecting telescope. Prior to Newton's work, telescope lenses refracted light (broke the light into its color components) which made looking at the heavens difficult. The Royal Society, purveyor of all the new sci-entific discoveries in England, asked for a demonstration, and Newton published his findings in a paper entitled "Optics." Society member Robert Hooke criticized some of Newton's findings. Newton was so offended that he withdrew from public debate about his work and counted Hooke his enemy until the man died.

Newton published a second tract on colors in 1675, but Hooke claimed Newton had stolen his ideas. Newton lashed out at Hooke again, and also vented his spleen at a group of English Jesuits who questioned his theories. Angry, formal correspon-dence between Newton and the Jesuits continued until 1678, at which time Newton sent one last furious letter, suffered a nervous breakdown, and then said no more. Newton's mother died the next year, adding to the man's anguish. He retreated into his laboratory for six years.

In 1687 Newton published the *Philosophiae Naturalis Principia Mathematica*, perhaps the greatest work on mathematics, physics and scientific method ever writ-ten, in which Newton laid out the three laws of motion. Newton did not discover gravity by observing a falling apple, but the great thinker did relate gravitational pull to elliptical planetary orbits.

Newton taught mathematics at Trinity College for many years but eventually grew tired of the students. He became warden of the Royal Mint in 1696 (England's version of Secretary of the Treasury). Newton's later years were devoted to his duties at the mint and study of the bible. He also served in Parliament. As Warden of the Mint he oversaw the "great recoinage," and when Newton rose to master in 1699 he took particular relish in pursuing counterfeiters and anyone debasing the currency.

Seeking counterfeiters in the taverns and brothels of London gave Newton a socially acceptable way to vent his rage, and he sent many to the gallows.

Newton served as president of Britain's Royal Society, whose members represented the best and brightest of the kingdom's scientists and researchers, from 1703 until his death in 1727. Queen Anne knighted Newton in 1705, the first scientist so honored.

Sir Isaac Newton presented a classic example of near-pathological imbalance. Although his latter years were marred by the grudges and jealousies he harbored against his fellow scientists, Newton never lost his faith in what he believed was the kernel of incontrovertibility in scientific method: the true north star of his own mental compass. Sadly, such a great man was rationally brilliant but emotionally stunted.

To achieve harmony, each one of the vital intelligences must develop through its own distinct stages:

- Physical intelligence grows from weakness, to strength, to power.

- Emotional intelligence evolves from a sense of "me," to "us," to a sense of "all of us."

- Mental intelligence starts with pre-rational (archaic, magical, and mythical thinking), then proceeds to rational thinking, and ultimately integral (integrated) cognition.

- Moral intelligence grows from selfishness, to caring for others, to concern for universal mankind.

- Spiritual intelligence includes one's own vibrational, energetic signature, our religious beliefs and meditative skills, progressing from fundamentalist, to liberal, to mystic.

Our peak development of each of these intelligences, blending them together in harmony, is the heart of body brilliance. Every person's peak level of brilliance is unique, dependent on the growth in each vital intelligence. The goal is not to master all the intelligences, but to strengthen those intelligences that are so weak they are causing problems. Author Wilber concludes, "For some this will mean clearing up a serious problem or pathology ... and for others, simply recognizing where their strengths and weaknesses lie, and planning accordingly."

FURTHER READING

Fadiman, James and Robert Frager. *Personality and Personal Growth.* New York: Harper & Row, 1976.

"Sir Isaac Newton." Available online at www.isaacnewton.utwente.nl/nieuw/ sir_isaac_newton/SirIsaacNewton.htm. Downloaded Jan. 2, 2005.

Wilber, Ken. "Introduction to Integral Theory and Practice." Integral Naked, 2003–2004. Downloaded January 2006. Available online: http://www.integral-naked.org.

*The curious paradox is that when
I accept myself as I am, then I can change.*

—Carl Rogers

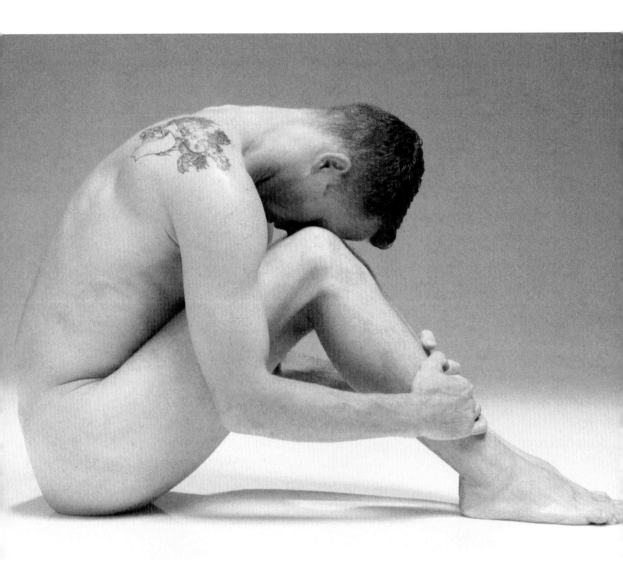

Chapter 5

The Power of Pause

Nature itself has a pulse, a rhythmic,
wavelike movement between activity and rest.
—Abraham Maslow

These early years of the new millennium, the twenty-first century, are heady, tumultuous times. In just five short years the globe has suffered heartbreaking death and destruction from wars, terrorist attacks, tsunamis, hurricanes, violence, environmental degradation, and hunger. Yet despite all this, spiritually committed people everywhere heed the call to brilliance in all avenues of life: business, government, health care, family, service. They—and we—answer the call to stoke the brightest lights of ourselves and greet each day with renewed effort to actualize our vital intelligences and bring peace and harmony to humanity. We are born for such times. We are called to fortify our truest selves, to direct our physical, emotional, mental, moral, and spiritual intelligences and shine them for all that is right and good in this world.

Whew! Although a most worthy pursuit, lifting the world (or just ourselves) out of darkness takes a lot of energy. I believe that we possess the brilliance to accomplish this task; that by living through our bodies' intelligences we can marshal our defenses—and offenses—and direct them toward the greater good. But if in our zeal to achieve these goals, whether personal or societal, we forget to take time to replenish our energies, we risk physical or mental collapse.

And in the scope of all the work needing to be done, it's easy to exhaust ourselves in the process—to run on fumes, or worse, flat out of gas. This is where practicing the simple "power of a well-intentioned pause" becomes a necessity. Type A workaholic personalities succumb to more health problems and risk sacrificing family and relationships for a very good reason: they don't value the power of pause.

The very nature of energy is to expand and contract. It's one of the few constants in the universe. The stars and their moons rise and set, waves of water crest and fall, electricity pulses, hearts contract and beat, lungs rise and fall, orgasms come and go. Energy may be constant, but it oscillates. The intelligences in our bodies are the same.

- Physically, we have times of effort and times of rest and sleep.
- Emotionally, we try to balance our sense of individuality and our need to connect with the people around us.
- Mentally, we can be muddled and confused, or focused and clear.
- Morally, we can pursue lives and ideals we don't truly want for ourselves, or we can exemplify our deepest values in the world.
- Spiritually, we can remain dormant, or we can sparkle and thrive.

Pausing—taking a break, a rest—rejuvenates the body and prepares it for the next round of exertion. We won't last too long without stopping to catch our breath. But in these times of overstimulation, hyperactivity, and multitasking (admit it: you drink, talk on the phone, and drive at the same time), our bodies consume tremendous amounts of energy that must be restored. If we are to thrive, seeking happiness through the harmony of our vital intelligences, we must learn to balance performance with rest.

Unplug yourself from the demands of your day and just stop for a few minutes. Take some deep breaths, try to clear your mind of all the chaotic details of modern existence, and focus on some place or event that was happy or beautiful. Sit quietly for ten minutes and relax. Don't worry; the kids, the telephone, the projects can usually wait for ten or fifteen minutes. You'll be amazed to discover that the project that seemed out of control before you took a break now seems more manageable.

Flavius Philostratus, an Olympic athlete trainer in ancient Greece, wrote about the importance of this "work/rest" ratio almost 2,000 years ago. More recently, performance psychologists Jim Loehr and Tony Schwartz tried to identify what separated the tennis superstars from the good players. Both were technically competent, often sharing similarities of stroke, speed, and ability to score. What they discovered is that the top players pursued a small personal ritual to calm their breath and heart rate *after* and *between* each point. These "well-intentioned pauses" might be as short as ninety seconds or less, but as techniques to focus the players' attention for the next stroke they were highly effective.

For the rest of us, however, a "power pause" of ninety seconds probably won't be enough time to rest and refuel. Relaxation novices need at least ten to twenty minutes to soothe frazzled nerves. Ask your colleagues, kids, or partner to respect your downtime; try to avoid answering questions or the phone. Don't be embarrassed by taking a break. We all need one. Unfortunately, most of us do little more than reach for the remote control at the end of the day, thankful to have survived another one. Relying on the tube alone to refuel your energies overlooks so many other means of healthy, fulfilling activities. Consider these suggestions for rest and relaxation:

- Simple exercise such as stretching, sit-ups or push-ups, even in your office.
- Walking, preferably outside, so you can enjoy the day.
- Taking a class in dance, yoga, or Tai chi for balance and movement.
- Calling a good friend just to talk.
- Savoring a meal, either alone or with friends.
- Eating lunch away from your desk, and taking your entire lunch period for lunch, not errands.
- Sneaking a nap.
- Getting a massage
- Luxuriating in a bath.
- Listening to music.
- Reading.
- Pursuing a favorite hobby.
- Praying or meditating.

Once you've added small daily breaks to your routine, why not take a full day? At least start with a half day. Too often the weekends seem like extensions of the work-week, full of errands and chores. Sometimes even socializing with friends becomes a hassle instead of a treat. Try spending an entire day at a park or beach with your family; walking the dog; enjoying a sport or hobby; taking a picnic out in the country, or dozing in a hammock while you pretend to read. Take time to talk to your family and listen when they answer.

Okay. You're ready to graduate to weeklong vacations and maybe even longer. People who boast that they haven't taken a vacation in years have not done themselves any favors. These longer pauses do not have to be car trips to ten different destinations or a week with the relatives. You're supposed to relax, not need a vacation from your vacation. Consider a retreat, a cruise—anything that refuels your energy, not saps your strength.

Author and spiritual advisor Deepak Chopra, M.D., maintains a grueling schedule of writing, workshops, and personal appearances, often working on four or five books at once and traveling frequently. To restore his equanimity he sets aside four to five weeks of vacation with his family, perhaps skiing or visiting sacred sites. But his most important rejuvenation practice is called *simran*, or total isolation—no books, telephones, magazines, radio, or any communication—for five to seven days, every three months, for reflection and meditation.

Closer to home, my friend Katy Caldwell is the director of Legacy Community Health Services in Houston, encompassing the Montrose Clinic and other medical services available to anyone, no matter what they can pay. Founded originally to test and treat those suffering from HIV/AIDS and sexually transmitted diseases in a nonjudgmental environment (the clinic is where I learned I was HIV-negative), the clinic now offers health counseling and wellness programs, in addition to more traditional doctors' visits and an in-house pharmacy. Katy works miracles every day to find financial support from businesses and the general community, as tightly stretched resources accommodate a growing clientele of the indigent and uninsured, no matter what their gender orientation.

Since late August 2005, the Montrose Clinic has become the primary medical provider for victims of Hurricanes Katrina and Rita. Over 150,000 refugees from Katrina alone poured into Houston, most without anything but the clothes they were wearing when they arrived. Staffers at the clinic have spent hours attempting to re-create destroyed medical records, get patients into counseling and patient services, set up doctors' appointments and dispense costly medications.

The needs of former and new patients—and finding the funds necessary to minister to those needs—never cease. But the escalated pressures of Katy's frenetic schedule have made it even more vital that she remember the power of pause and take time for herself. Besides receiving massage therapy, Katy disappears into a spa every now and then. Working out the physical kinks helps realign her thinking as well. Katy would not be the only loser if she didn't acknowledge the importance of downtime.

In *The Power of Full Engagement*, energy management expert Jim Loehr spells out the need for taking a pause:

> *After a period of activity, the body must replenish fundamental biochemical sources of energy ... Increase the intensity of the training or performance demand, and it is necessary to commensurately increase the amount of energy renewal ... Balancing stress and recovery is critical not just in competitive sports, but in managing energy in all facets of our lives.*

The point at which an object's weight balances perfectly on a base is called a fulcrum. The most obvious example is a playground seesaw; the beam rises and falls on its point of equilibrium. Hanging artwork on the wall requires finding the fulcrum of the wire, or otherwise Uncle Thaddeus appears a bit tipsy. Determining the fulcrum varies by the weights of the two sides; if one side is heavier, that greater weight must be shifted toward the fulcrum to regain the perfect balance point.

Finding equilibrium in one's life—determining the point of balance between activity and rest—is more difficult than hanging a picture. We Americans, in particular, steeped in the work ethic of our Puritan forefathers, seem to feel guilty if we are not completing a Herculean task in record time. We don't procrastinate well.

But all our attempts at harmonizing the vital intelligences will fail unless we stop and rebalance work and play, set limits, and distinguish between "hard-charging" and "recharging." In other words, we have to find the fulcrum that equalizes our active lives with our downtime so that efficiency doesn't end in burnout. For some people, that well-intentioned pause could require a "force" of will. If that describes you, make the effort.

I used to run myself ragged, starting my day at 5 a.m., staring at the computer, and finally dragging home by 9 p.m. after a long day of teaching and clients. I filled my days helping others find their way to brilliance and trying to raise my own levels of vital intelligence through bodywork and exercise. But by the time I stumbled through the door I was too tired to talk or eat. I longed for personal time and time to share with my partner Jim.

So I took back my time, vowing not to forget the benefits of a well-intentioned pause. My new schedule, enhanced by strategic pauses throughout the day, allows me to come home ready to enjoy my partner and our evening together. Such time is like a mini-vacation. I'm convinced I accomplish even more with less aggravation.

Whether you decide to take a six-month sabbatical or just expand your lunch period to a full hour, you are acknowledging the body's need for rest and rejuvenation. Go ahead, make your escape. Or as a woman in a bath-soap advertisement said as she sank into the tub, eagerly anticipating the bliss of a bubble bath, "Calgon, take me away."

Visit www.BodyBrillianceBook.com to download more examples of "well-intended pauses," or better yet, post your own favorite pauses.

FURTHER READING

Loehr, Jim, and Tony Schwartz. *The Power of Full Engagement: Managing Energy, Not Time, Is the Key to High Performance and Personal Renewal.* New York: Free Press, 2003.

2

LIVING THROUGH YOUR BODY

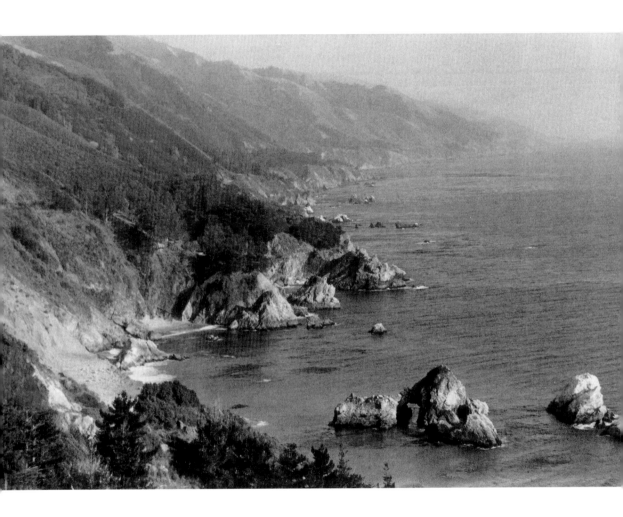

CHAPTER 6

Rancho Strozzi

*We are arriving at one of the most fruitful and
important turnings in the history of the race.
The self is entering into relation with the body.*
—Edward Carpenter

Petaluma, California, March 1994: My rental car rolled along Middle Two
Rock Road in the glorious California sunshine, with the backseat stuffed with
luggage and groceries for the long weekend. Petaluma, an hour's drive north
of San Francisco, lay a few miles behind me. I savored the crisp March air breezing
in through my open car window. It was a welcome change from Texas's humidity
and heat. The road crested and I stopped to enjoy the view: a valley of rock forma-
tions, farmhouses, and sheep in just-greening pastures. I love this part of California;
its beauty and isolation speak to me—so different from my hometown Houston, a
sprawling city of concrete and glass. With a deep breath I realized just how good it
felt to be there.

I continued my drive to Rancho Strozzi, a lovely place with grazing horses and
buildings of weathered wood. My assigned cabin was tucked away behind the martial
arts dojo. Once inside, I chuckled. The cabin, charmingly rustic, was a tall but small
octagonal room with a loft just large enough for a mattress. There was a wood-
burning stove for heat, a small refrigerator, a sink, and a round table with one chair.
Windows opened out onto the surrounding fields of hay. Only the occasional gust of
wind broke the blissful silence.

An hour later I was back on Highway 1, cautiously maneuvering the hairpin
curves, until with a dip and a wide turn, the rocky hills finally revealed the coast.

Thrilled with excitement, I drove on for a while, splitting my attention between the road and the spectacle of ocean before me, then parked and sat as close to the rock's edge as I dared. In wonder, my eyes were riveted to the ocean below me: the towering cliffs, the boulders jumbling out to the sea below, the play of light changing the color of the water. The waves roared far below with the constant frigid blow of the Pacific wind. I'd always loved the ocean; I used to rent an apartment in Galveston, on the Gulf of Mexico, but this stretch of the Pacific was the most beautiful I'd ever seen. Feeling calmer, I returned to Rancho Strozzi and settled in, ruminating on this day and how I came to be here, and anticipating my start at the Lomi School the next morning.

The year 1993 was a breakdown year for me. Richard Strozzi-Heckler says, "When life breaks down, break through." It's his twist on, "When life gives you lemons, make lemonade." The year before, two friends of mine, lovers David Arpin and Mikel Reper, and I opened a business. Mikel dreamed of opening an aromatherapy gift store. In those days, aromatherapy—the use of essential plant oils—was bursting into popularity. I dreamed of a massage clinic and day spa, a center where all my fascinations converged: hands-on healing, face and body care, exotic baths and muds, meditation and Tai chi combined with aromatherapy. We agreed that a little vegetarian sandwich shop would be a nice addition to the mix. The vegetarian food would accent the healing arts and attract people to our business.

We rented a grand old house on West Alabama in Houston's museum district. Never mind that the building had seen a series of failed restaurants and bars. Our friend Craig (Ms. Craig Ann we called him) joined us as kitchen manager. Mikel and I consulted a Buddhist psychic and feng shui master, who made suggestions on color schemes, which doors to use, and blessed our business to ensure its success. After twelve years of bartending to the fabulous, I resigned to build a career in the healing arts, confident in our venture.

The Enchanted Garden opened in March 1992. The aromatherapy store was a big hit, and my private massage practice flourished. People loved the vegetarian restaurant, too, but it was expensive to operate. The spa, however, with seven treatment rooms, never succeeded well enough to keep all the therapists busy. And conflict began even before our opening. Mikel's and David's relationship was unraveling, and they were soon in divorce court—or as close as two gay lovers could get. It wasn't long before David and I spent as much time and energy managing Mikel as we spent running The Enchanted Garden itself. David and I, willing to be fair and generous, cut Mikel ample slack, but after a year tolerating his alcohol and drug problems, an intervention, and rehab, we finally cut Mikel loose.

Unfortunately, by then our enthusiasm, momentum, and finances had suffered permanent damage. Ms. Craig Ann, bored with the conflict and politics, quit. David, a health care consultant, was on the road during the week and returned to the Garden to work weekends. That left me to supervise the spa, the restaurant, and the aromatherapy store through the week. By October 1993 The Enchanted Garden was insolvent, the victim of our own poor management and underfunding, and David and I, exhausted, closed the business. We lost our investment and then some, and I was saddled with more debt than I could have imagined. (David says ours is the most expensive friendship he's ever had.)

The Garden was a success on other levels, however. I did have a solid massage practice that supported me well. When the Garden closed I moved the remnants of the spa to an office building on Richmond Avenue near Greenway Plaza. Essential Touch, like a phoenix, rose from the ashes of The Enchanted Garden. I had learned many hard and valuable lessons on how to run a profitable and professional business.

Meanwhile, as The Enchanted Garden spiraled to its demise, a more devastating loss cut my heart: my dear friend, Michael Mosley, was dying. Michael and I, along with Jon, Ms. Hill, Bobby, and Harry were the foundations of the "gang," or more accurately "the girls": about thirty guys who traveled in a large pack to concerts, the bars, movies, dances, and just about anything that was fun while overindulging in drugs and alcohol. Michael and I were especially close as we had similar tastes in music, movies, the arts, and architecture. Having both worked in the club scene for years, we understood the trials and tribulations of a bartender's life.

By 1993 we had seen the ranks of our gang destroyed by AIDS. Of the thirty-plus guys who played, partied, and loved as friends and sometimes boyfriends, there were ten of us left. Jon, J. D. and myself are the HIV-negative ones. Ed, Robby, Danny and his Robby, Bill and Trent, Joe and Michael, Bobby, Ronny, Art, Ms. Ricky, Tessy, Phyllis, Gavin, Jeff, and the others had died, one by one, whittling our numbers down. And now Michael was dying too.

Michael had wasting syndrome, which reduced his once-rugged good looks (he was a magazine cover boy) to skin and bones. His face had become a skeletal mask. He had no energy. I had to shout to be heard, as his hearing was gone. One of the last things we did as a group was see Bette Midler in concert. Michael needed help getting dressed, then we escorted him, step by painful step, into the Summit Arena for the show. He couldn't hear a thing, but he insisted on seeing the Divine Miss M and going out with the girls one last time. Friends were scattered throughout the audience, and as we waited for Bette they came over to say hello and pay their respects to Michael one last time.

By January 1994 Michael had been admitted to Twelve Oaks Hospital, and on a cold January night I went over to visit. Faking a warm hello to the receptionist, I thought about how many times I'd ridden this elevator car to the AIDS floor and wondered again why I had remained healthy, potent, and alive when so many had dwindled away in pain. Utterly helpless, I stood outside Michael's room, trying to muster up a thin cheerfulness before I entered. Michael lay quiet but alert as I kissed him on the cheek. His mother, Mary Lou, busied herself with little chores, and Jon (aka Cha-Cha), Michael's roommate, sat near the bed. In hushed whispers he filled me in: "He can go anytime. Dr. Rios says there's nothing else to be done."

My usual chatty cheer, however strained, vaporized in the inevitability of my friend's death. I had no words. So I did what I have always done: I went to work, offering Michael a foot rub. He mumbled his assent as I pulled up a chair, grabbed some coconut lotion, and untucked the sheets. I began with the right foot, gently pushing, pulling, and rolling. As I rubbed, pressed and stroked his feet I conjured all the love I felt for this man and pooled it in my breaking heart. As I continued, I feebly directed my love through my hands into his feet and to his heart, and silently thanked him for all the fun and friendship we'd shared. But I did not cry. I haven't cried for years. As I finished with his left foot, Michael gave me a cold look and pulled both his feet up toward his butt, signaling he'd had enough. I visited for a while longer then said good night, kissing Michael on the cheek as I left.

It was late and I felt weary to the bone. I debated whether to turn off the ringer of my phone, as I always did, finally deciding a full night's sleep was more important than the sad news I was expecting. When I woke up the next morning, my mind still tired, the light on the answering machine blinked. Sure enough it was Jon, telling me, "It's all over. Michael died peacefully about 3 a.m. Call when you can." I sat motionless; Charlie, my Burmese cat, sensed my despair and hopped lightly onto me. I petted him absentmindedly as he licked my hand, eventually curling up in my lap. I sat, unmoving, with Charlie for a long time, until I had to shower and go to work.

With Michael's death I vowed that 1994 would be a turnaround year for me. I was utterly depressed: we had lost the Garden, I was nipple deep in debt, Michael died, and I weighed 320 pounds, at least a hundred pounds too much for my height and stature. I had to do something radical to change my mood and regain a sense of my life.

One day my friend and massage teacher Ann Lasater was reminiscing about the Lomi School, where she went in the late 1970s. Four friends, Robert Hall and Richard Strozzi-Heckler and their ex-wives Alyssa and Catherine, founded the school about 1970. They were the first to synthesize psychotherapy, breathwork, bodywork, movement, and meditation into a cohesive method. (Lomi is a Hawaiian style of massage, but the word "lomi" was chosen for the school because it means "to touch.")

Offhandedly Ann remarked that Robert Hall, one of the founders of the school, was gay. In all my years of studying spirituality and human potential, I'd met only a few gay men. They, like me, were novices on their path. Incredibly I now learned that Robert Hall was gay too. He was no novice, however, but a pillar in the transformational community: a psychiatrist and an assistant to Fritz Perls, the co-founder of Gestalt psychology. Robert was one of the first Americans to learn Ida Rolf's bodywork system of Rolfing. Later, traveling in India, he met Dr. Randolph Stone, the founder of polarity therapy, and brought him to California to teach.

I *knew* I had to study with Robert Hall. It took a few months to make the necessary arrangements. I combined all my debts with the Consumer Credit Bureau and agreed to a monthly payment plan. Included in my living budget was the cost of the Lomi School tuition. My friend David Arpin, with lots of frequent flyer miles from his travels as a health care consultant, graciously agreed to trade facials for ten airline tickets to San Francisco (he still has beautiful skin).

But now, outside Petaluma, all the pieces had come together. Here I sat, nestled on a cliff, savoring the spring sun and biting Pacific wind, and anticipating this next stage of my life. When I first sat down I felt tired and weary with grief, but an hour later my heart was lighter (although my cheeks stung with the cold). Acute gratitude for life's generosity temporarily replaced my sorrow, and I sensed a familiar longing to follow the advice of an old advertisement: to be all I can be.

Even after conquering the AIDS demon, embracing sobriety and turning my life around, I was buffeted by the loss of friends and financial security. And my body suffered as a result, making recovery much more difficult. As the sun and wind comforted my soul, I dared to hope that through the Lomi bodywork I could learn how to shine again. Maybe I could squeeze lemonade from life's lemons. I would soon find out.

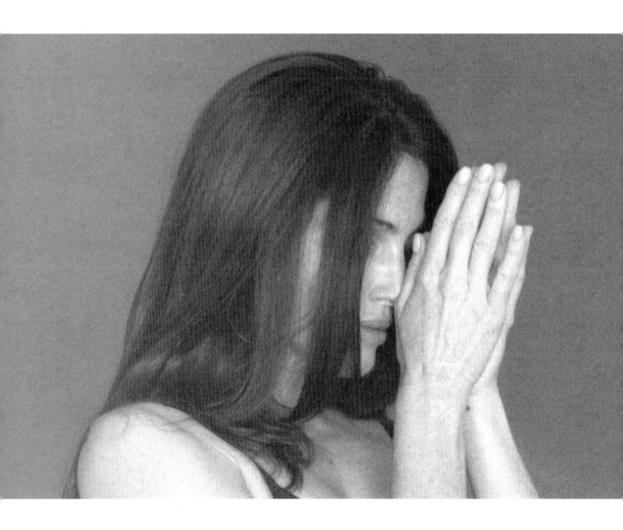

CHAPTER 7

The Lomi School

*Lomi work [is] ... demanding of people. It asks that
people wake up—wake up to their bodies and their lives.*
—Robert Hall

Rancho Strozzi, March 1994: The next day dawned spectacularly. I snuggled warmly under layers of blankets, yet my visible breath confirmed that the fire in the cabin's small stove had died out hours ago. I lazed for a few more minutes, anticipating the shiver of throwing off the covers and dreading the thought of the unheated outdoor shower. With the precision of a military campaign I launched out of bed, built a roaring fire, started the coffeepot, and braved the colder outdoors. The cabin was toasty hot by the time I returned from my freezing, yet oh-so-invigorating shower. Satisfied with a breakfast of fruit, cereal, and coffee, I went to the aikido dojo and waited for the others to arrive.

The dojo is divided into three rooms. The largest is stretched with padded mats for classes, and there is a small sitting area with couches and a rough-hewn kitchen. Twenty-one students gathered with Robert Hall and Richard Strozzi-Heckler that morning, and the two men outlined our time together, saying that:

- The Lomi School teaches somatics: a body-centered way of living.

- We will use bodywork, breathwork, yoga, aikido movement, and sitting meditation to bring attention to our bodies.

- These disciplines are taught as ways of working toward physical vitality, emotional stability, and personal effectiveness.

- This focus on the body develops awareness and self-acceptance. It allows us to know ourselves more fully—how we stand and breathe, how we express our emotions, how we perceive the world, and experience it.

- Group process is the primary tool we use to explore the edge of our fears and leave the comfort zone of our everyday lives; to share the stories of our hearts; to develop trust and community; and to support each other in self-discovery.

- Lomi work also explores how social activism grows from self-discovery and our connection to the social issues of our time, "including birthing, dying, conflict resolution, education, violence, community, the arts, and health care."

After presenting a short overview of the training, Robert and Richard wanted to hear from us, asking, "Who are you? How did you come to be at the school? What do you want from our year together?" Richard took notes as we introduced ourselves. I tuned in as the first of my classmates shared, but I didn't hear much. As usual, I felt shy and anxious about telling my story. I realized that I wouldn't hear anything about the others if I didn't raise my hand and give my own introduction. I remembered my vow to make 1994 different, and why I'd traveled so far to be here, in this dojo, with these teachers. Normally I would wait until the last to share, but now I seized the moment and raised my hand.

With a Southern drawl I nervously introduced myself, telling tersely of Ann Lasater's teaching and how she was my inspiration to be here, about my depression, the close of my business, Michael's death, crushing debt, being gay, and David's generosity with the airline tickets. It took just a few minutes to cover the basics, and I was deeply relieved as the spotlight shifted to the next person. My breath calmed and my listening sharpened as I quietly celebrated my little victory.

We were a diverse group: a police lieutenant and a paramedic, an arch Democrat, other massage therapists and chiropractors, a psychic, psychotherapists, students and teachers, a carpenter, and a director of nonprofit organizations. We agreed to meet for nine weekends throughout the year and a weeklong retreat in July. Some of us were there for our professions, but we were all there for ourselves.

At the break we mingled and ate delicious pastries from the Tomales Bakery on Highway 1. Still feeling self-conscious, I cautiously visited with my classmates and won the prize for coming the farthest distance. Some of them had traveled for several hours to get there, but I was the only non-Californian. I remembered that California is as long as Texas is wide. Thankfully, my classmates welcomed me, and I began to relax and feel more comfortable with the group.

With the preliminaries over, I looked forward to participating in the Lomi School's regimen of bodywork, exercise, meditation, and group process. I was convinced that Robert, Richard, and the class would help me heal my depression and all the sadness of my recent life. As you will see, I still had much to learn.

But first, if I am going to show you how to peak your vital intelligences to achieve body brilliance, I need to discuss how perceptions of our bodies have changed over time and the theories and techniques surrounding that metamorphosis.

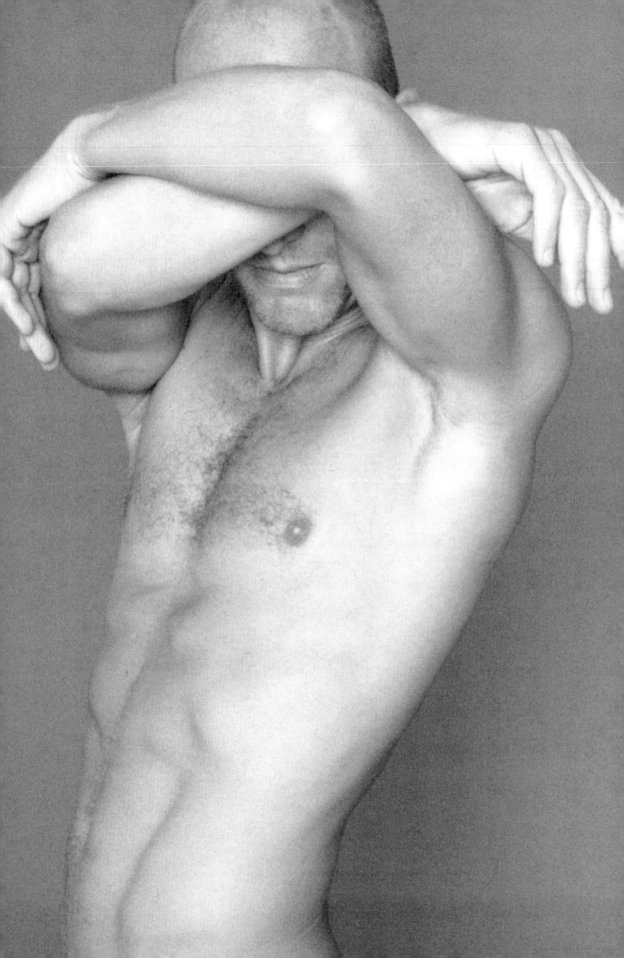

CHAPTER 8

The Living Body

*The great mystery of the world is not the
invisible, but the visible.*
—Oscar Wilde

Western civilization has not been kind to the human body. The past 2,400 years have seen the body worshipped, debauched, vilified, denied, ignored, and mechanized. The ancient Greeks celebrated the human body, glorifying it in art, sculpture, and athletics. The philosopher Socrates taught that the supreme understanding of beauty started with the body: through the body a transcendent understanding of beauty and the virtues of all life itself was achieved. The Greek Olympic Games were the ideal test of physical strength, endurance, and mental and spiritual purity.

With the dawn of the Piscean age power shifted to Rome. The Romans absorbed much of Greek culture, including body worship. (Celtic warriors, however, who always went into battle totally naked, terrified the Roman legionnaires.) But by the third century of the Common Era, Christian bishops targeted the drunken debauchery and sexual excess associated with pagan Roman festivals initially for sublimation into church-approved celebrations and eventually for total elimination. Church fathers portrayed the body as carnal, gross, and prey to base appetites for 1,700 years, convincing the faithful that sex and pleasure were to be avoided, not celebrated. The seven deadly sins of greed, lust, gluttony, pride, anger, sloth, and vanity would not even exist without the body. The road to heaven lay in transcending the body, an idea common to most of the world's religious and mystical traditions, not just Christianity.

French mathematician and philosopher René Descartes delivered another "body blow" when he declared, "I think, therefore, I am." Descartes' statement defined the Age of Reason, placing emphasis on the mental intelligence at the expense of the other intelligences and reducing the body to a crude bundle of organs and nerves that supported the intellect. Modern medicine, with its trove of technology, doesn't treat the body much better, often seeing it as an object—even a project—to be poked and prodded, analyzed and diagnosed, rather than as the physical manifestation of a person.

Somatics, on the other hand—the focus of study at the Lomi School—is a body-centered approach to living. The Greek word soma means "living body." In ancient India, Brahmin priests drank a hallucinogenic concoction called *soma,* named after the Vedic god Soma, in rituals to expand consciousness. Richard Strozzi-Heckler defines "somatic" as "the living body in its wholeness; or mind, body and spirit in unity."

The idea that the body itself had value, alone or in concert with the mind, resurfaced in the twentieth century. In particular, the relatively recent blending of Western psychology and medicine with Asian philosophies dramatically shifted the way we viewed and experienced our bodies. In traditional Western thought, the connection between body and mind was "psychosomatic," which referred to health problems caused by distress or other manifestations from the mind (it's all in your head). Many Asian cultures, on the contrary, saw the body as the very foundation of health and spiritual life.

The Lomi School was the first to synthesize different approaches of body-centered therapies into one curriculum. The importance of attention, or focus, lay at the center of Lomi proficiency, but the ideas of Wilhelm Reich, Fritz Perls, and Asian training in meditation and aikido also influenced the method. Additionally, Lomi co-founders Robert Hall and Richard Strozzi-Heckler borrowed from Randolph Stone's polarity therapy and the structural massage work of Ida Rolf.

The tenets of the Lomi School can be summarized as follows:

- Vitality, in the form of energy currents, flows through every body; when that vitality is fully realized we experience a natural state of health and well-being. If our vital energy becomes clogged or blocked, we experience disease.

- Somatic exercises, principally concentration or attention, strengthen the body, charge the spirit, and relax the mind.

- A relaxed mind is interested and engaged in the present moment, with a tender attention to subtle change—not just differences in the body, the ebb and flow of emotions or fleeting thoughts, but to the laws of change that govern life and the world we live in.

- The primary goal of somatics is the union of body, mind and spirit: to achieve harmony outside oneself by finding harmony within.

Wilhelm Reich (1897–1957), known as the grandfather of somatic psychoanalysis, was an Austrian psychiatrist trained by Sigmund Freud in Vienna. In 1922, Reich established a private practice in psychoanalysis as part of Freud's Polyanalytic Polyclinic, where he researched the social causes of neuroses (early psychoanalysis focused on personal neurotic symptoms).

Reich came to believe, however, that a person's entire character or personality could be examined and treated. Reich's first book, *Character Analysis,* outlined his theory, called "ego psychology," and started a small revolution in psychoanalysis. Reich also discussed what he called "body armoring": the theory that unreleased emotions, especially those related to sexual energy, actually produced "armor," or blocks in the muscles and organs, and became stored in seven parts of the body—eyes, jaws, neck, chest, diaphragm, belly, and pelvis—preventing the release of energy. Reich believed that orgasm as part of a healthy, mutually satisfying sex life was one way to break through the body armor—a seemingly simple solution that initiated a great deal of controversy among his peers. During the 1930s Reich also claimed to have found the physical energy *orgone,* which he said was contained in the atmosphere and in all living matter.

The Nazis banned Reich's second book, *The Mass Psychology of Fascism,* in 1933. German newspapers branded him a Communist Jew who advocated the dangerous idea of "free love"; fearful for his life, Reich emigrated to the United States to continue his orgone research. Unfortunately, Reich did not escape harassment in America. In 1947, following a series of articles about orgone in *The New Republic* and *Harper's,* the U.S. Food and Drug Administration (FDA) began an investigation into Reich's claims about orgone therapy, and won an injunction against its promotion as a medical treatment. Charged with contempt of court for violating the injunction, Reich conducted his own defense, which involved sending the judge all his books to read. He was sentenced to two years' imprisonment. In August 1956, several tons of his publications were burned by the FDA. He died of heart failure in jail just over a year later, one day before his parole hearing.

Fritz Perls (1893–1970), a psychiatrist and student of Reich's, helped found Gestalt Therapy. *Gestalt* in German means "an irreducible experience," and Perls adopted the term to name the method he had developed with his wife Laura, also a psychiatrist. Their approach emphasized the person as a whole—with the mind and emotions equally connected to the body—which differed from the importance of "knowing" stressed in Hans-Juergen Walter's Gestalt Theoretical Psychotherapy.

Perls theorized that the exhilarating experience of living fully alive, aware, and in the present was actually derailed by our habitual thinking mind. ("I think, and that gets in the way of who I am"—apologies to Descartes.) Our thoughts about life created a barrier to experiencing life full tilt, and Gestalt therapy emphasized the removal of obstacles that prevented people from maximizing their potential. The method involved working in real time as opposed to focusing on past experiences, the norm for psychoanalysis. His 1951 book, *Gestalt Therapy: Excitement and Growth in the Human Personality,* also featured contributions from Paul Goodman, an anarchist and political writer, and from Ralph Hefferline, a psychology professor and patient. Perls was quoted as saying, "Lose your mind and come to your senses."

The key points of Gestalt therapy are:

- *Live now,* in the moment.
- *Live here,* in the present.
- *Stop imagining,* and experience reality.
- *Stop unnecessary thinking;* decide and act.
- *Start expressing* and avoid manipulating, explaining, justifying or judging.
- *Stop restricting awareness* and accept unpleasantness.
- *Resist* accepting "should" or "ought" from others.
- *Begin taking full responsibility* for actions, feelings, and thoughts.
- *Begin surrendering* to who you are right now.

Claudio Naranjo, a Chilean-born anthropologist and psychiatrist, organized Gestalt therapy into three basic principles:

- *Actuality:* nothing exists outside the present moment.

- *Attention:* awareness of feelings, thoughts, body posture, breathing rhythm, physical sensations, sights, sounds, tastes, smells, and so forth to enhance day-to-day experience.

- *Responsibility:* taking full responsibility for your own actions, feelings, and thoughts.

In addition to his work with Gestalt therapy, Naranjo experimented with mind-altering substances and was a major figure in the Human Potential Movement and the Fourth Way.

Perls, meanwhile, became associated with The Esalen Institute in California in 1964. People who had no connection to psychotherapy often recognized Perls as the author of a 1969 quotation described as the "Gestalt Prayer":

> I do my thing and you do your thing. I am not in this world to live up to your expectations, and you are not in this world to live up to mine. You are you, and I am I, and if by chance we find each other, it's beautiful. If not, it can't be helped.

Ida Rolf (1896–1979) obtained her doctorate in biochemistry in 1920. By the mid-1950s Rolf had developed a method for realigning the human structure in relation to gravity, originally called the Structural Integration of the Human Body but commonly referred to as Rolfing. The Lomi School curriculum included Rolf's bodywork program because it provided an excellent way to break up the emotional armoring in the muscles and connective tissues by employing deep-tissue massage. These techniques realigned the body's posture, muscles, and bones.

According to Rolf, bound-up connective tissue or "fascia" restricted opposing muscles from functioning independently from each other. She claimed she could separate the bound-up fascia by separating the fibers manually through her technique and then re-engaging effective movement patterns. Adequate knowledge of living anatomy and hands-on training were required, Rolf said, in order for a practitioner to safely negotiate appropriate techniques and the depths necessary to loosen the bound-up fascia.

Rolfing involved a series of ten bodywork sessions. The therapist photographed the patient's body before the first session, assessing posture and imbalances. Each session focused on a different part of the body, with the first session devoted to the chest in order to open and relax the patient's breathing. Next the therapist worked to build a solid "foundation" by focusing on the feet, ankles, and legs. Once these stabilized the therapist turned to the pelvis to create a solid base for the torso and arms. Later the head was "put on straight." Final photographs revealed the changes in posture. You could see, as well as feel, the physical benefits of this work. After the muscles, tissues, and bones had settled for a period of time, the patient could schedule five advanced sessions or the occasional "tune-up."

As Ida Rolf worked with people, she discovered a link between muscle tension and suppressed emotion. When muscle tension was released, she found that some people experienced "flashback" memories of the original situations that first caused the need to tense the muscles. A sudden release of the trapped emotion cleared the need for the tension to be held by the tissues. As a result, Rolf said, the body returned to a more natural posture. Both The Rolf Institute and the Guild for Structural Integration continue to teach Rolf's method, and many other groups that offer deep-tissue bodywork trace their lineage to Rolfing.

The fourth major bodywork program adopted by the Lomi School, polarity therapy, concentrated on the energetic grid of the body and relieving blocks in it.

Dr. Randolph Stone (1890–1981), the founder of polarity therapy, emigrated to America as a youngster around 1898. He completed his primary medical certifications in the early 1920s, including as a doctor of osteopathy, a doctor of chiropractic and doctor of naturopathy, but he was a lifelong student, eventually adding certifications in a wide range of topics including massage and midwifery. His love of travel took him in search of medical insights from other cultures. The good doctor maintained a medical practice in Chicago for over fifty years, where his motto of "Whatever works, works!" established his reputation for taking otherwise hopeless cases, many of whom responded to his unconventional techniques and multicultural approaches.

Endlessly curious, Stone was fascinated by spiritual studies and mysticism. In the 1940s he deepened his knowledge of and commitment to esoteric understanding by accepting initiation in a meditation system based in India. His dedication to this yogic path continued uninterrupted for almost forty years, and he made frequent visits to India to study and develop his inner knowledge.

By the late 1940s Stone had synthesized his collected information into his first book, *Energy*, published in 1947, theorizing that the polarized fields of attraction and repulsion, as found in all magnetic relationships and in the atomic substructure, were the underlying reality of all physical phenomena, especially health. A series of seven books and pamphlets followed, further explaining his basic ideas about energy and providing numerous healing techniques.

In the mid 1950s Stone tried to interest the medical community in his ideas, offering free lectures, writing journal articles, and repeatedly attempting to engage his colleagues in dialogue. These efforts were largely unsuccessful, as medical professionals from that era confidently pursued the miracles of drugs and surgery that characterized Western treatment.

In the 1960s, already in his mid-seventies, Stone suddenly found popularity for the first time with a new generation of health seekers for whom his blend of science and spirituality was not so unpalatable. In seminars in California he vigorously preached his message of holistic health. The seed of polarity therapy finally found enough fertile soil to survive. Dr. Stone retired in 1974 and moved to an Indian meditation community, where he offered free medical services in a public clinic. He gradually withdrew from public life, dying of natural causes.

Besides the above therapies, the Lomi curriculum featured the Asian ways of aikido, Hatha yoga and Vipassana sitting meditation. Aikido, developed by Morihei Ueshiba, is a Japanese martial art for self-defense that harnessed universal love to heal conflict, create fluidity of the body, and strengthen personal energy. *Aikido* was often translated as "the way of spiritual harmony." This translation pointed to a practitioner's skill at controlling an attacker by redirecting his energy rather than by blocking an attack. (See the anecdote about aikido and emotional brilliance in Chapter One.)

To understand this skill, visualize the way a flexible willow bends with the storm, whereas the stout oak breaks if the wind blows too hard. Ueshiba taught that the principles of aikido should be applied to every aspect of one's life, and he once remarked that he was teaching students not how to move their feet but how to move their minds.

In the West, the term *yoga* is associated with the stretching postures of *Hatha*, one branch of India's classical spiritual disciplines. Most Western yoga classes had little or nothing to do with Hinduism or spirituality, but were simply a way of keeping healthy and fit. Traditional Hatha yoga was a complete yogic path, including moral disciplines, physical exercises (e.g., postures and breath control) and meditation, encompassing far more than the yoga of postures and exercises practiced in Western physical culture.

Yoga lovers see daily practice as beneficial in itself, leading to good health, emotional well-being, mental clarity, and joy in living. Yoga adepts progress towards *samadhi,* a high state of meditation and inner ecstasy. For the average person still far from enlightenment, yoga can be a way of increasing one's spiritual awareness. While the history of yoga strongly connects it with Hinduism, yoga lovers claim that it is not a religion itself, but contains practical steps that can benefit everyone.

Vipassana, which means "insight," was a body-centered meditation technique attributed to Buddha.

Vipassana, often called *mindfulness* meditation, focused on the many sensations and feelings of the body. Meditation calmed the mind and strengthened concentration. The mind was able to "stop and see" (remember the power of a well-intentioned pause in Chapter Five?), ready to receive the spirit's insight. In this calm centeredness, the practitioner gained knowledge of whatever disturbed his mind, which led to pure wisdom and eventual healing. Followers of Vipassana eliminate the desires and emotions of greed, anger, and ignorance that corrupt the mind.

The last century of the millennium ushered in a valuable shift in the way we humans experience our bodies, yet in many ways our physical selves remain a mystery. For many women, the intricate interdependence of their complicated systems remains uncharted territory. It is a recent phenomenon for women to demand control of their physiology and anatomy. But for men or women, our bodies are the only concrete reality we can know. They are always with us, constant, living and breathing in present time. Our bodies never lie, and with careful stewardship they will reveal all the secrets leading to truth. And when we work to achieve body brilliance, mastering our five vital Intelligences, our bodies shine.

As Lomi founder Robert Hall noted to me, "Enlightenment is, after all, a bodily process."

Visit www.BodyBrillianceBook.com to read more examples of somatic pioneers, or better yet, post your own favorite body/mind teachers.

FURTHER READING

Fadiman, James, and Robert Frager. *Personality and Personal Growth.* New York: Harper & Row, 1976.

Hanna, Thomas. *Somatics.* Reading, MA: Addison-Wesley Publishing, 1988.

Harvey, Andrew. *The Essential Gay Mystics.* Edison, NJ: Castle Books, 1997.

Perls, Fritz. *Gestalt Therapy: Excitement and Growth in the Human Personality.* New York: Delta, 1951.

Reich, Wilhelm. *Character Analysis.* New York: Noonday Press, 1962.

Stone, Randolph. *Polarity Therapy: The Complete Collected Works.* Reno, NV: CRCS Publications, 1986.

Somatic: the living body
in its wholeness; or mind, body,
and spirit
in unity.

—Richard Strozzi-Heckler

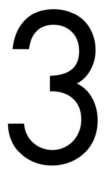

3

PHYSICAL INTELLIGENCE— THE FIRST VITAL LAYER

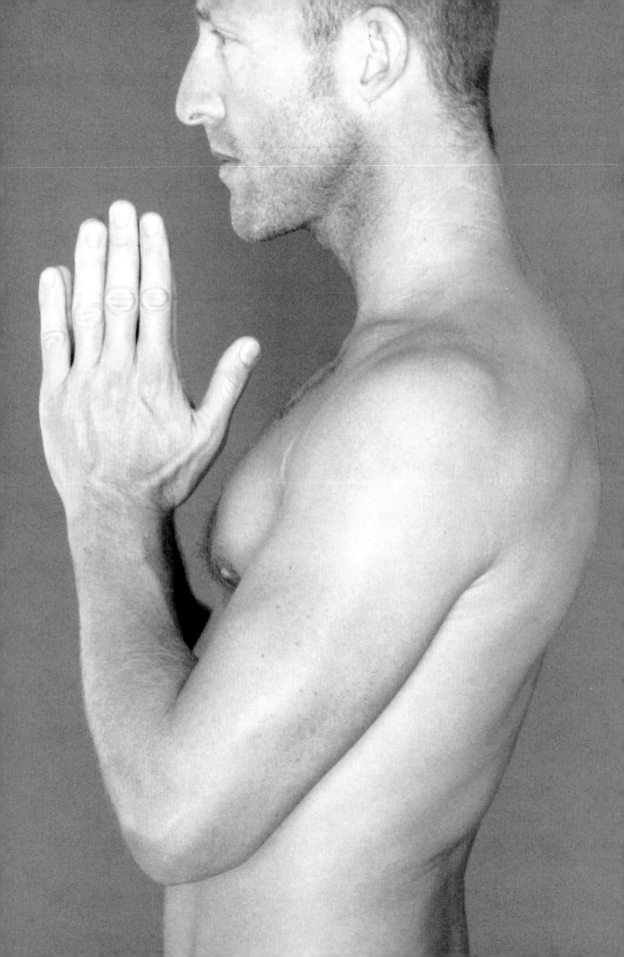

CHAPTER 9

Bones, Muscles, and Joints

You should meditate on how it is
that the soul loves the body.
—Meister Eckhart

Torino, Italy, February 2006: Representing China at the Winter Olympic Games, Zhang Dan and her partner, Zhang Hao, stepped onto the ice for their free-skate performance. They ranked second after their dazzling performance in the short program, and since the pair skated last, the silver and bronze medals were still very much in play. The young couple's skating is punched by their power, speed, and grace. The Zhangs (they are not related) are famous for their quadruple twist, a very difficult maneuver during which Hao spins Dan four times as her body is almost horizontal and parallel to the ice.

A few seconds into their program, they attempted something never before tried in Olympic competition: an unprecedented quadruple throw salchow, in which the man throws his partner into the air as she launches from the back edge of her skates, spins four times, and lands gracefully on the ice. As the crowd gasped, Zhang Dan missed the graceful landing. She crashed, her left knee slammed into the ice and her legs splayed out. Dan spun across the ice and rammed into the sideboards surrounding the rink.

Visibly stunned and doubled over in pain, Dan struggled to her feet with her partner's help. Hao held her gently from behind, as they glided to the sidelines, seemingly finished. Five minutes later, after consulting with coaches, a medic, and officials, twenty-year-old Dan gingerly returned to the ice. The crowd roared and she even managed a timid smile. The pair continued their performance to the thundering applause of the crowd.

No one could have expected much from Zhang and Zhang after such a shocking accident. I can't imagine what high demands are placed on all the elite Chinese athletes, or what Dan's life has been like to create this kind of sheer willpower. "We are challenging the extreme limits of what a human being can do," said Zhang Dan. "We were still empty in our minds. When the music started again we didn't know where to start our elements, but we gave a gesture and then we carried on." Hao added, "Gradually after we restarted, it became more clear in our minds how we could continue."

Following a display of bravery seldom seen on an ice rink, the Zhangs began again and nailed every move. Four minutes later, the entire crowd was standing and cheering their effort, which gave them second place and China's first-ever Olympic figure skating silver medal. By the time they came out to receive their medals, Dan's left leg was heavily iced and bandaged. The plucky skater, however, limped a victory lap around the rink to still more applause.

Through training and sheer will Zhang Dan and Zhang Hao mastered their physical intelligences. They were ambassadors representing the four qualities that make up this vital intelligence: strength, flexibility, grace, and bearing.

Houston, Spring 2004: The stained glass windows in my studio were flung open on a crisp spring day. I was dressing the massage table for my next client when I heard the faint sound of laughter. My third-story, walk-up studio was near Woodrow Wilson Elementary School, and I had a bird's-eye view of the playground from my bathroom window. It sprawled over an entire half block along Fairview Street. Kids were out for recess doing what kids have done for recess since the Dark Ages, or at least since I was a kid in the 1960s. I paused at the window to enjoy the sights and sounds of kids playing and having fun.

Two teams of kids scampered across the grass playing kickball. Three girls added giggles of delight to their cartwheels. Phys-ed teams leaped like frogs, racing each other to a finish line; the winning team let loose with a whoop. A gang of girls practiced cheers, stacking themselves into a human pyramid and laughing when it fell down. The playground could have been any circus, with the acrobats wearing red or blue school uniforms instead of colorful sequins and feathers. The breeze carried the sounds of squealing, happy children.

I pondered a mystery of life. Sometimes I still wonder why I was in such a hurry to grow up. Somewhere along the way the carefree play of children shifted to the march of adulthood. We traded running, jumping, and tumbling for walking, standing, and sitting. Instead of crawling through bushes like kids, as grown-ups we lean against watercoolers. Rather than stomp around the great outdoors, we sit at our desks for too-long hours. We trade glee for the safety of our paychecks.

At a certain age we began to really slow down. The normal movements of our every day suddenly caused a dull ache that often, over time, spasmed into full-blown pain. We attributed these accumulating aches and pains to "getting old." We resigned ourselves to the march of time without ever asking, "Does it have to be this way?"

The answer is, "No, it doesn't." I don't believe in "getting old," per se. I believe that with our minds focused on the daily rat race, our bodies simply forget how to feel alive and free: a classic case of "You lose what you don't use." Those once-young and limber bodies have become tired and brittle.

One natural antidote to the ravages of time is to realize consciousness throughout the body's five vital intelligences. A somatic life empowers a man or woman to live with a relaxed and concentrated mind, a strong, flexible body, and with sparkling, mature emotions that enable that person to share his/her love with others. It is a life that is dynamic, creative, and harmonious. The bedrock of this vital life is our physical intelligence, the first layer of consciousness. The physical intelligence is the densest of the five layers so that it can provide a stable foundation. It includes our muscles, joints, and bones, as well as the connective tissues: the tendons, ligaments, and fascia.

This level of our gross anatomy allows us to stand upright and to move, twist, turn, walk, and bend. Our fundamental experience of health and our sense of well-being depend on the vitality of this layer. Fitness experts have long recommended we use at least three different types of exercise to reach full physical health, including muscular fitness and flexibility, aerobic and endurance fitness, and techniques to lower the percentage ratio of body fat to muscle.

The four chapters covering physical intelligence are Strength, Flexibility, Grace, and Bearing. I think of them as the four pillars of our body's foundation. The Zhangs, the amazing Chinese Olympic skaters profiled above, have these qualities in spades. But each of us can peak these proficiencies to our best abilities and grow this layer of intelligence.

The coastal soil along this stretch of the Gulf of Mexico near Houston is reclaimed swampland: layers of wet clay, rocks, and dirt. Here in the Montrose, a neighborhood near downtown, many of the old houses are built on pier-and-beam foundations. Large pillars are sunk deep into the earth and rise vertically above the ground's surface. Beams are fastened horizontally to the pillars to create a stable foundation, one that can provide equal stability during long, hot summers and cold, wet winters. The house is then built on top of the pier-and-beam structure.

Like the old foundations in Houston, the four pillars of Strength, Flexibility, Grace, and Bearing, working in harmony, create a dynamic platform for our body's physical, emotional, mental, moral, and spiritual health. Chapter Ten, "Strength," covers the importance of building our muscles, followed by a discussion of conscious calisthenics in Chapter Eleven. "Flexibility," Chapter Twelve, explains the importance of stretching and the body's full range of motion. "Grace" in Chapter Fifteen covers our joints, balance and coordination. And Chapter Sixteen, "Bearing," explores good posture and the natural position of our bones and how the muscles and connective tissue supports or distorts them. This chapter also explores the effects of touch and deep-tissue bodywork on this layer of intelligence.

The exercises for peaking this first layer of intelligence are like many exercises found in the physical fitness canon. They focus on building muscle strength and endurance, stretching, and balance. In most physical fitness programs there is an emphasis on mindless repetitions or laps. The difference with somatic exercise is the attention given to the raw experiences of our body as we exercise. The intention is not only to build muscle strength, flexibility and balance, but also to unify those skills with our feelings, thoughts, and soul. The more our attention is engaged during these exercises, the greater our experience and the benefit.

Read about the different exercises for fitness and increasing your vital physical intelligence. Think about how you can design a conscious exercise program that works best for you. Start as easy as you like. My best reason for doing anything in life is to feel good, or better yet, to feel great. The point of living through your body is to enjoy yourself day in and day out, NOT to suffer through agony to finally arrive at happiness, or enlightenment, or something, somewhere, sometime in the future. Feel better now.

The important goal of any fitness program or spiritual practice is to stick with it. Play around with the different exercises to see which ones you like and that work for you. The following five-step program is good for anyone, whether you're doing high-intensity training and sports competitions or just an easy workout.

- Warm up with any light aerobic exercise, like a brisk walk, easy jog, bike ride, or swim.

- Do some warm-up stretches (see Chapter Fourteen for some good examples).

- Proceed to your high-intensity workout, which could be vigorous sprinting, regular calisthenics or the Five Tibetans (see Chapter Twelve).

- Start a warm-down with any light aerobic activity like those suggested for the warm-up.

- End with deep stretches like those in traditional Hatha yoga.

You will notice good changes if you commit to just fifty minutes for your routine: a ten-minute walk, ten minutes of light stretching, ten minutes of whatever high-intensity work you want to do, ten minutes of warm-down aerobics, and ten minutes of deep stretching. You can start with less and add more minutes as you progress.

Next, set a weekly goal of how often to do the exercises. Decide how many days you can really do your routine: two, three, four times a week. Start modestly and work up to more exercises and more days when it feels good to you. It is better to consistently meet your simple goal of a few exercises a couple of times a week than to occasionally do a longer and more vigorous program, one you can't or won't maintain.

As you live through your body, improving your five vital layers of intelligence, you will feel the echoes of your childhood vitality start to bubble up. Let your longing for a brighter and healthier life pull you forward. If you get discouraged, just remember that your mind gives up long before your body does, so keep going. You can do this.

I will address aerobic fitness and the ratio of body fat to muscle as part of my dis-cussion of the second layer of vital intelligence, covered in the next book of this series.

FURTHER READING

Deuster, Patricia A., ed. *The Navy SEAL Physical Fitness Guide*. Old Saybrook, CT: Konecky & Konecky, 1997.

Leonard, George. "Towards a Balanced Way." *The Lomi Papers*. Mill Valley, CA: The Lomi School, 1979.

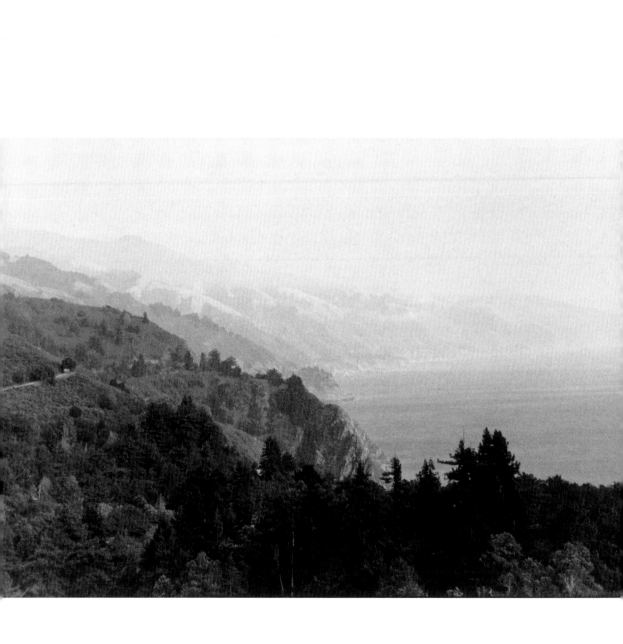

CHAPTER 10

Strength

Those who think they have no time for bodily exercise will sooner or later have to find time for illness.
—Edward Stanley

Petaluma, California, July 1994: Struggling thirty-five feet in the air, I tried to reach the platform above me. I was only halfway up the pine tree, and the rope ladder proved a rascal to climb. Unattached at the ground, it twisted and turned as I tried to climb it. My breath was labored, and my arms were tired. I rested a moment, my arms woven through the ropes. The ladder bent almost ninety degrees as my weight forced my feet straight out from my arm hold. I wasn't scared of falling, exactly, because I was strapped to a safety belt that was anchored by four of my teammates on the ground. I had some small concern that my 300 pounds (I'd lost twenty pounds since the training began) will uproot my teammates if I should slip, but I expected they could handle it.

Our guide up on the platform gently encouraged me to keep climbing. My team, below me on the ground, shouted their encouragement as well. I untangled my arms and pulled myself up another rung. My progress was slow, but I was climbing. My energy stalled a few feet from the platform as my arms trembled from what seemed a Herculean effort to pull my weight this far into the sky, almost seventy feet up now. I wove my arms through the ropes to rest one more time. I didn't know if I could climb another rung. I thought, "I will hate myself for giving up," but I was exhausted. My arms, back, and legs ached. The four rungs to the platform seemed like a mile. I focused my attention on my breath to calm my mind, and with a last-ditch effort I summoned a glimmer of energy and climbed the last four rungs. Apparently, the mind gives up before the body does. I was so grateful to feel the solid wood platform under my arms. Our guide helped me to swing my legs onto the perch, while the entire team let loose a raucous cheer seventy feet below me.

I quietly gloated to myself. Finally, mind triumphed over matter; my willpower was stronger than my "fat" body. Now I stood to face the next challenge: grab a handheld trolley, step off the platform, and ride a cable across an open meadow to the ground. I could hear the ocean off to my right. Richard stood on a ladder across an open field at the base of the cable. I had been so focused on scaling the rope ladder that I forgot to dread stepping off seventy feet into space.

My guide deftly disconnected my safety belt from my teammates on the ground and strapped me to the hand trolley. I stepped up to the edge. Fear gripped my belly and tightened my throat as I looked at the ground, my teammates tiny in the distance. What the hell? This has got to be easier than climbing that damn ladder. Before I can think about it any more I stepped off. The fear immediately gave way to the blast of shooting down the cable. The thrilling sensation was better than any roller coaster. I shot past Richard on the ladder and hurtled toward the tree that anchored the cable. My momentum slowed, and I swung back toward the ground. With a few swings back and forth, Richard grabbed me from his post on the ladder. I was breathless with my feats and proudly declared to him, "I can never call myself a sissy again." Richard promised, "I'll bear witness to that."

Houston, July 2004: It was 7:30 in the morning, and I was plastered again. I don't mean plastered in the usual sense of "way too many beers," but plastered as in soaking wet, of every fiber of my clothes drenched in sweat. I was halfway though an hour of military-style maneuvers. My chest was heaving from a vigorous blend of calisthenics and running/walking. Welcome to SEAL Physical Training (PT), the exercise (some might say torture) program developed by a former U.S. Navy SEAL (Sea, Air and Land).

"Wide-grip push-ups," called the instructor, "Twenty of them. Starting position. Ready! One, two, three," he droned. "One," we completed the four-count chant. "One, two, three," he repeated. "Two," we counted the reps. The count volleyed until we reached the magic finishing number of twenty.

With just a millisecond to breathe, the instructor barked, "Close-grip push-ups, twenty of them. Starting position. Ready! One, two, three," started the chant.

"One," we called back. And so it went as we worked our way through a series of chest exercises, abdominal workouts, tricep dips on the bleachers, step-ups using the benches of picnic tables. I was momentarily relieved when he called for a run/walk (how tragic is that—who would have thought?). "Intervals, at your own pace. Two laps."

SEAL PT in Memorial Park is the brainchild of Jack Walston, the former Navy SEAL. Walston created the exercise program to give civilians a taste of military physical fitness. Each class is led by a crack former military instructor—a U.S. Army Ranger, a U.S. Navy SEAL, a Navy medic, a couple of marines.

There are two levels of entry: Boot Camp and Body Camp. Boot Camp is a two-week intensive, some might say exhaustive, mental and fitness training program. After finishing Boot Camp graduates may choose to continue in the ongoing "Lifers" program. The "Lifers" workout at 5:30 a.m. is intense (I would say grueling) and doesn't leave time or energy for socializing.

Body Camp is billed as a four-week workout for those too injured or out of shape to complete Boot Camp. Body Camp graduates can join the "Navigators," designed as an ongoing, easier program. I opted for the Body Camp, and it was hard work. And to my surprise, I liked it.

What a turnaround. I took two years of Air Force ROTC in high school so I could skip the required phys-ed classes, partly because I felt embarrassed about my body and partially because I hated the exercises. As a kid I did like to hike and ride horses when we lived in the country, but overall I was lazy. I would just as soon watch TV or read as to exercise. After years of neglecting my body I was disgusted with it. When I reached a weight of 320-plus pounds, when climbing a flight of stairs left me winded, I realized that if I was ever to be fit and trim (which I'd always dreamed of) exercise would have to become my friend.

In December 1997, I went to visit my good friends Creighton Edwards and Michael Fife at their home. Both are regular massage clients. Creighton is an internationally respected surgeon. Once after an angioplasty he asked me to come to the hospital to deliver some aromatherapy oils for his sutures and give him a reflexology foot massage. I wasn't about to miss a surgeon asking for natural treatments in addition to his hospital care.

As I was leaving he asked me to come to his house to give him a massage, noting that he wouldn't be able to drive for a few weeks. When he felt a bit better I went to their home. As I said my hellos I met their three dogs: Willie, Waylon, and Hank. Hank was a half-greyhound mix.

Later, as I was winding up the massage with Creighton, I was holding his feet, feeling the energy move through me and nurturing his body. Suddenly the voice that I sometimes hear at the back of my mind said to me, "Adopt a greyhound." This came as quite a surprise to me. I hadn't had a dog since the seventh grade. I considered myself a cat person, although my last cat, Charlie, had disappeared.

The more I researched greyhounds, the more I thought I could live with a dog like that. They are beautiful, they are quiet, and they are loyal and affectionate. And they need to be walked regularly—not just let out into the yard but actual exercise. Greyhounds are athletes, after all. I also knew to trust my voice.

Two weeks later, just a few a days before Christmas, I brought home a handsome greyhound. We started exploring the old Montrose neighborhood, walking from Miramar Street to Hermann Park, or we'd cut across to North and South Boulevards. Every day we explored new routes. I loved being out in the cold of winter. Alexander, a handsome fawn color, looked smart in his black jacket, collar, and leash.

One morning a few months later, Alexander and I were out walking, and I heard the voice in the back of my mind again. This time it said, "Ask Gary to work out with you. Get a trainer."

It was no surprise to me when Gary Archer, my old friend, said, "Great idea." In a few weeks I joined the Downtown YMCA, and Gary and I had a trainer and a regular workout program. Our trainer, Mary Hodge, was a nationally ranked mountain biker. After a few months of working with her I dusted off my bicycle and started riding.

As I began to see pleasing changes in my body, that positive reinforcement led me to maintain an exercise regimen. My program has ebbed and flowed along with my weight, but I keep coming back to exercising my body.

Eventually I changed trainers and gyms. Alvin Reuben, my new trainer, is a massive, handsome black man and a former pro football player. I wanted the results I saw in his body and the clients he trained. He also worked carefully with my back injury, a chronic condition I had suffered with for years. Alvin's method of training requires the mind to perform the exercise, slowly and carefully, and let the body build its strength naturally. Master the movement and you carefully build the body. With Alvin's technique, weight lifting became a meditation. Every exercise began with my body relaxed. I would use light weights and attentive focus and breathing through each movement. Under Alvin's firm gaze he would stop me if I lost control of the exercise, or if I sped up to use momentum rather than my strength. Using Alvin's technique in the gym turned working out into a spiritual practice.

Through those years I lived with a compressed spinal disc in my back, a chronic pain that would sometimes flair up with excruciating spasms. For the most part I just lived with the discomfort, but after a long bout of chronic pain I took a few months off from the gym to nurse my back. Not surprisingly my weight began to rise without regular exercise.

My friends Gibbie and Marlene are SEAL PT Lifers. They met at SEAL PT and later married. I had always blown off the whole boot-camp-and-exercise-at-5:30-in-the-morning thing. When Marlene was ready to return to SEAL PT after Emily, their daughter, was born, she opted to start with the Navigators, which met at a more civilized 6:30 a.m. I was intrigued as Marlene described the easier pace and lighter attitude. I wasn't sure I could even handle Navigators with my back, but knew I wanted to try something different. So there I was, my clothes plastered to my body on a hot and humid July morning.

I was shocked that I liked SEAL PT. But most surprising was my back. I was very careful with the exercises; I did as many reps as I could and would rest or modify the movement when my back started to hurt. The overall calisthenics strengthened my back, which in turn greatly reduced the pain.

Ironically, strengthening my abdominal muscles—my bid to strengthen my back—had overdeveloped my hip flexor muscles. Your abdominals, or abs, are the four layers of muscle that span your sides and belly, from the lower rib cage to the hip and pubic bones. Strong abs are important for good back support and good breathing. (The more toned and supple your ab muscles, the deeper your breath exhalation, which in turn gives you a fuller inhalation. This simple improvement in breathing alone yields a dramatic improvement in vitality).

The hip flexors are the muscles that raise the thigh up toward the belly. Some of the hip flexors attach to the back along the lumbar spine. My overly strong hip flexor muscles had actually strained and pulled the lower vertebrae out of alignment, and this miscalculation had caused much of my back pain. The remedy was to focus on strengthening the back muscles themselves and ab exercises that counter-strengthened the hip extensors: the muscles that lift your thigh backward and up.

I had never worked as hard in my life as I did in the SEAL PT Navigator program. But I liked the challenge and felt slow, often achingly slow, progress. I was getting stronger and my stamina improved. Marlene said it took about six weeks for the body to acclimate to the intensity of the workouts.

As I jogged along through Memorial Park that July morning, I recalled how it had taken every ounce of energy I could muster to conquer that platform and hand trolley ten years earlier. Now here I was, enrolled in a Navy SEAL workout program, and I was actually enjoying it. Even calisthenics, the bane of high school gym classes, had become an invaluable part of the development of my physical intelligence. As the slogan said, I'd "come a long way, baby." And all these efforts provided the added benefit of mending my aching back. I smiled to myself as I contemplated this amazing turn of events.

On the journey I became at home in this marvelous creation of a body and actually began to love my body, imperfections and all.

For those of us that believe in a creator, how better to connect with that force than through the body— the crowning creation according to Genesis?

—Dave Allen

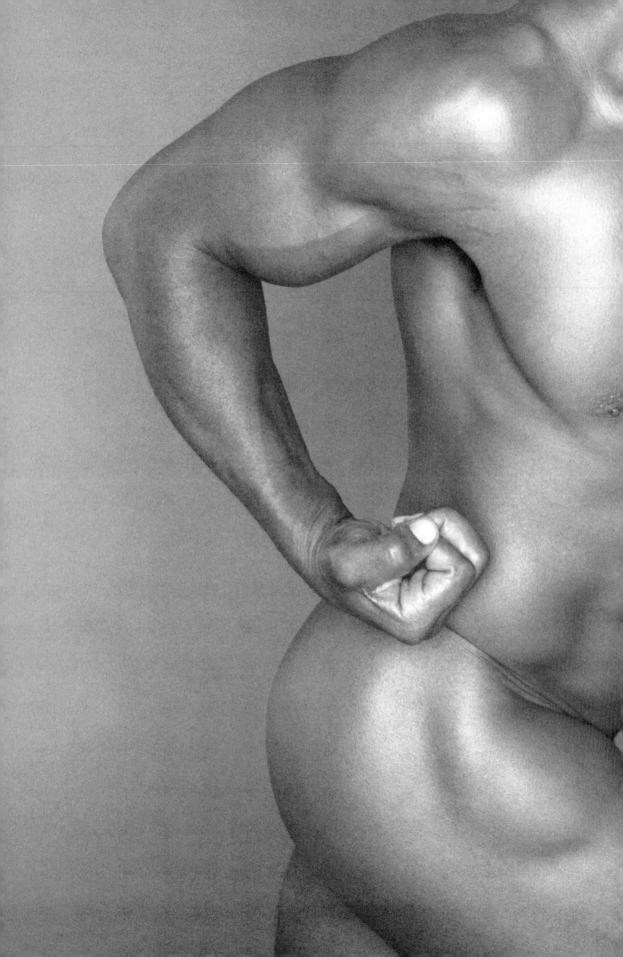

CHAPTER 11

Conscious Calisthenics

A bench press is little more than an upside-down push-up ...
and a lot less convenient.
—Kristofer Hogg

My years in the gym and as a massage therapist have taught me the importance of strong healthy muscles, and I knew I wanted to include "working out" in *Body Brilliance*. SEAL PT showed me that any park in the world is a potential gym; picnic tables, bleachers, jogging trails, and sandy volleyball courts can all be used to strengthen muscles and stamina.

"Calisthenics" comes from the Greek words *kallos* for beauty and *thenos* for strength. These healthful exercises are designed to create muscle fitness, which includes muscular strength, gracefulness, and physical well-being. Calisthenics, as they are taught in traditional physical education classes, can be boring and usually have a bad rap. I am amazed that I enjoy the SEAL PT workouts so much—that I'm paying good money to enjoy what I avoided (what I considered pure hell, actually) in high school.

Muscle fitness refers to both muscle strength (how heavy an object you can lift) and muscle endurance (how long can you lift it). Keeping our muscle strength is important for good health. Every pound of muscle we have burns thirty-five to fifty calories a day. And as we age most of us lose one pound of muscle mass a year. This weakening of the muscles leads to the loss of normal strength, balance, and coordination.

Compare calisthenics to the two most popular forms of exercise: weight training and aerobics. Aerobic exercises are running, biking, brisk walking, and swimming. According to *Yoga Journal,* aerobic exercise is anything that raises your heart rate to at least 55% of its maximum (the highest rate you can maintain during all-out effort is generally estimated at 220 minus your age). Calisthenics aren't usually done fast enough and long enough to have a full aerobic effect, although some of the SEAL PT instructors deliver an intense combo of running and phys-ed drills; I often feel I've gotten my aerobic workout. Conscious calisthenics, with their focus on slow breath and movements, do not qualify as an aerobic exercise.

Weight training is done to build bigger and stronger muscles. In a gym, with proper weight machines, you can easily isolate the muscles you are training and adjust the weight of the exercise. With calisthenics you are limited to the weight of your body, for better or worse. Once you reach peak performance with calisthenics you can't gain extra strength without going to a gym. But most folks aren't even strong enough to lift or pull their own body weight. A regular push-up requires your arms to raise and lower two-thirds of that amount. Use alternative exercises to build the muscles strong enough to support the body's full weight.

A great way to gauge your muscle fitness is the "day-after effect." And what is that? Knowing your body intimately is one of the goals of a somatic life. We've all felt soreness the day after engaging in some intense work or exercise. That soreness is usually attributed to lactic acid buildup in the muscles. Lactic acid occurs naturally as a chemical by-product of muscle exertion. Once the lactic acid builds up to the point of pain, it takes the muscle tissues a few days to flush out the excess acid. Since the day-after effect is an internal gauge, you don't need an expert or gadgets to measure your muscle fitness. But the day-after effect may be more than just the burn you feel after doing too many push-ups. More importantly, it serves as a guide to how hard you can push your body.

Product information for the HoloBarre, a super-strong metal bar that attaches in a doorway and adjusts within a track to accommodate different exercises, refers to the day-after effect as the "delayed onset of muscle soreness," or DOMS. DOMS is described as the actual increase of motor neurons (nerves) due to vigorous movement. Out-of-shape people, or even athletes after several weeks of lazing around, lose important neurological control of the muscles. With inactivity the motor neuron functions decline. The day-after ache of the muscles is actually the muscle fibers increasing their neurological activity. Even under very mild stress, muscle damage occurs, separating the fibers and damaging the cell membrane.

My twist is to combine the trainer Alvin Reuben's slow, conscious movements with traditional calisthenics. It takes more strength and control to do these calisthenics meditatively than to rush through them. The key is to slow down and use your breath as a guide. Match your movements to slow inhalations and exhalations. Breathe in to a slow count of four, and breathe out to a slow count of four. As you gain strength, you can slow down even more—inhale and exhale to counts of six or eight or ten as you move. Whether you are working out in the gym or the great outdoors, consciously slowing down your breathing transforms your exercises into meditations.

Conscious calisthenics becomes an ideal form of weight training. The difference between somatic exercise and other training methods is the attention given to the raw experiences of our body as we exercise. It is also far safer than weight lifting, which too often relies on rapid and jerky movements, which stress the body and can result in muscle strain and pain. Acute attention to proper body mechanics and super-slow movement through somatic exercise almost totally remove the risk of injury. This approach also increases the actual load, and thereby buildup, of the muscles being worked.

Super-slow weight training isn't anything new. Bob Hoffman, founder of the York Barbell Company, sold weightlifting courses as early as 1927 that involved very slow training speeds: reps with a ten-second positive and a ten-second negative. He also urged close attention to the beginning changes of each repetition.

Recently, Ken Hutchins, a former trainer for Nautilus exercise equipment, revived interest in SuperSlow training. Back in the 1970s, Hutchins worked with elderly women in an osteoporosis clinical study. Osteoporosis is also known as brittle-bone disease. He felt that the traditional speeds of lifting were too fast for such frail patients. So Hutchins used his slower lifting speeds with great results. Encouraged by the progress of the women, Hutchins began using SuperSlow training with people of all ages and abilities.

On the next few pages I cover some of the exercises, listed below, that exemplify conscious calisthenics, but this principal can be applied to almost any fitness program:

- Push-Ups
- Diamond Push-Ups
- Bench Dips

- Bicycle

- Ins and Outs

- Hindu Squats

- Walking Lunges

The key is to feel your body as you move slowly. Most phys-ed exercises are slammed out in a hurry. People rely on speed's momentum to carry them through the exercise, where the end result is more important than the journey. Conscious calisthenics emphasize just the opposite. By slowing down your movements and focusing your attention on breathing, you strengthen your muscles safely and with less pain. The ultimate benefit from conscious calisthenics is the experience of shaping your body and your life in a radical new way.

Visit www.BodyBrillianceBook.com to download your free written copy of these exercises.

FURTHER READING

Deuster, Patricia A., ed. *The Navy SEAL Physical Fitness Guide*. Old Saybrook, CT: Konecky & Konecky, 1997.

Some ways of working with our bodies …
can be taught so that a person can develop his or her
sensitivity to experiences of toning, stretching, and
vigorous effort, coming to a fuller knowledge
and appreciation of oneself.

—Unknown

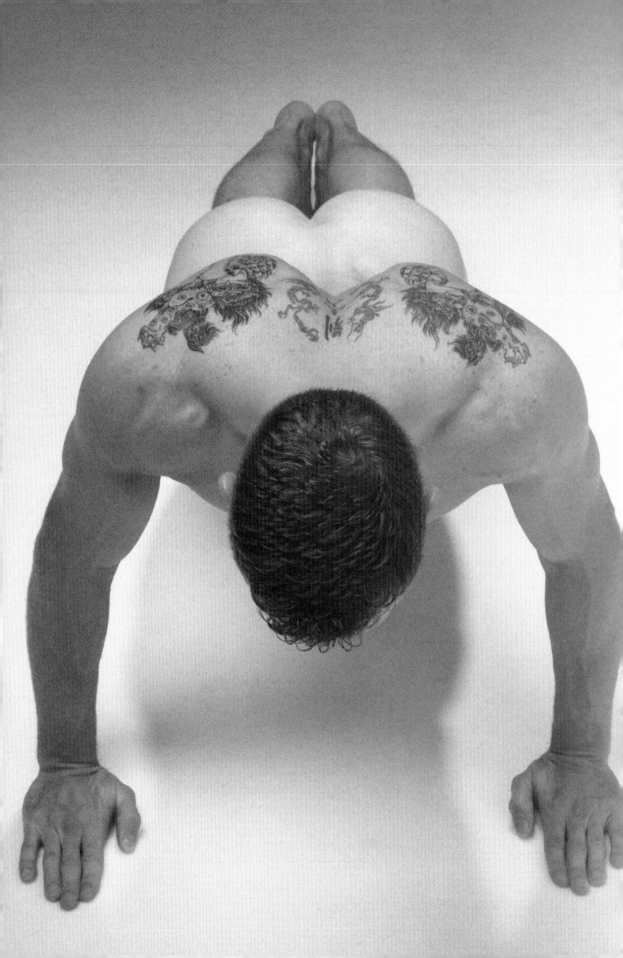

Push-Ups

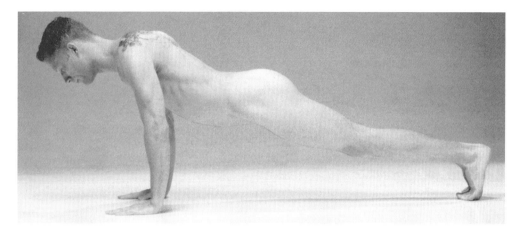

Lie facedown on the ground and curl your toes up so that you rest on the balls of your feet. Rest your hands alongside your chest, palms down.

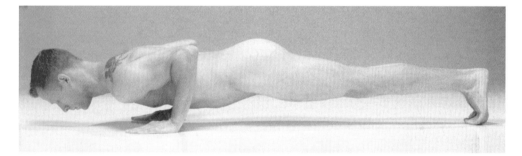

Tighten your muscles. Your head, back, glutes, legs, and ankles form an even plank. Breathe in slowly, straighten your arms, and lift your body up. Finish inhaling and pause just before your elbows lock.

Slowly breathe out and lower your body, maintaining your even plank. Your chest hovers four to five inches above the ground (the thickness of a water bottle) as you finish breathing out (exhalation). Repeat ten times.

To modify: Drop your knees to the deck. You can also push up on an incline, placing your hands on a table or bench. The angle allows for greater ease and range of motion as you use your strength for the push up. You can even press against a wall; this is called a push away.

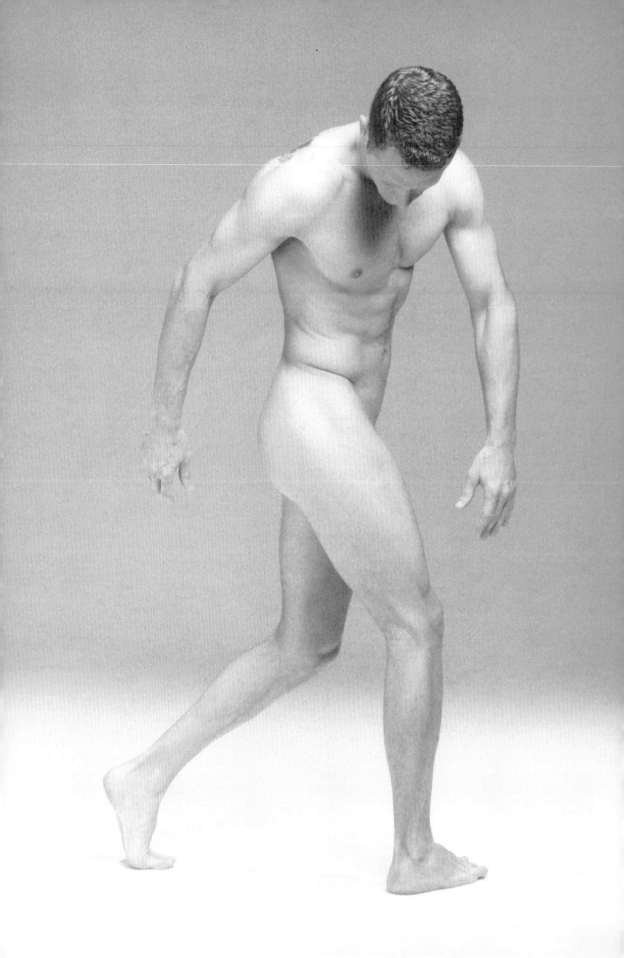

Diamond Push-Ups

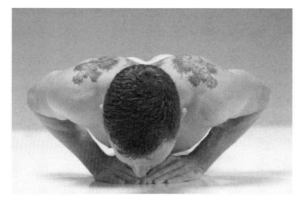

Your thumbs and index fingers touch to form a diamond as your hands rest under your chest.

Tighten your muscles. The head, back, glutes, legs, and ankles form an even plank. Breathing in, slowly extend your arms, lifting your body up.

Finish breathing in (inhalation) and pause just before your elbows lock.

Slowly breathe out and lower your body, maintaining your even plank. Your chest hovers four to five inches above the ground (the thickness of a water bottle) as you finish breathing out (exhalation).

Repeat ten times.

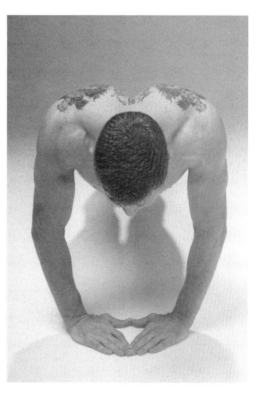

To modify: Drop your knees to the deck. You can also push up on an incline, placing your hands on a table or bench. This extra angle allows for greater ease and range of motion as you use your strength for the regular push-up. You can even press against a wall in a push away.

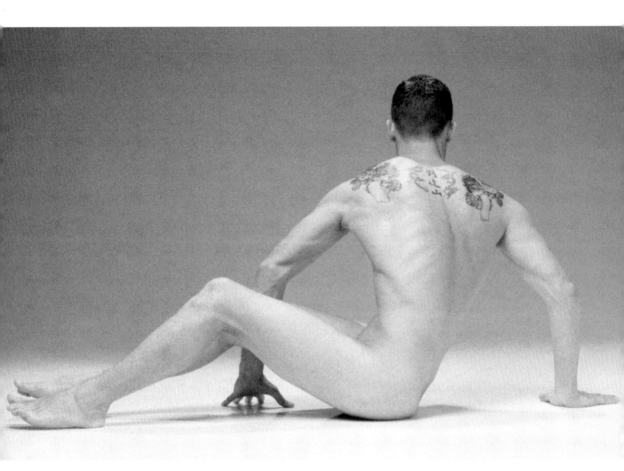

Bench Dips

Sit on the edge of a sturdy bench as your hands rest by your sides. Grasp the bench firmly, extending your legs fully with the toes pointing toward the ceiling (keep them active during the exercise).

Taking a deep breath, lift your hips off the chair as you slightly bend your arms. Feel the sensation of your weight being supported on the heels of your hands. Pause.

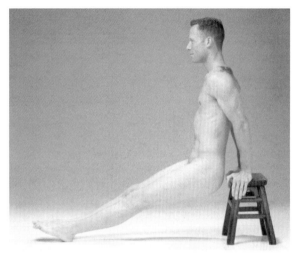

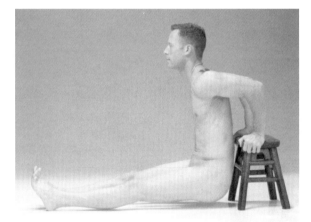

Breathing in slowly, bend your arms until the elbows are in line with your shoulders. This drops the hips below the bench.

Pause.

Breathing out, slowly push yourself back up. Pause.

Repeat twenty times.

To modify: You can bring one foot or both feet flat to the ground. This lightens your weight to give extra support.

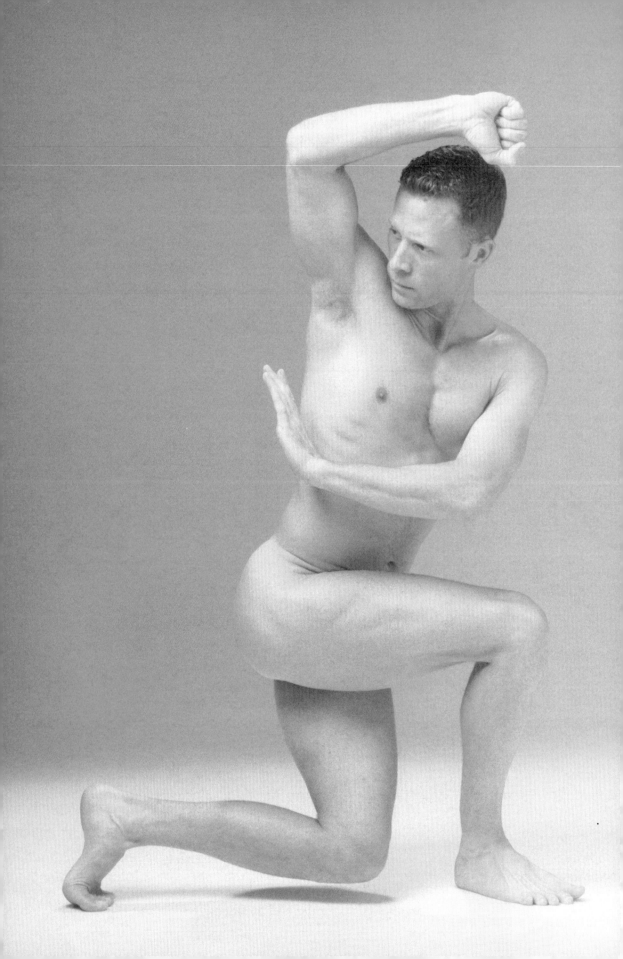

Bicycle

Lie on your back with your fingers interlaced behind your neck or head. Your knees are bent with the thighs forming a ninety-degree angle to your body.

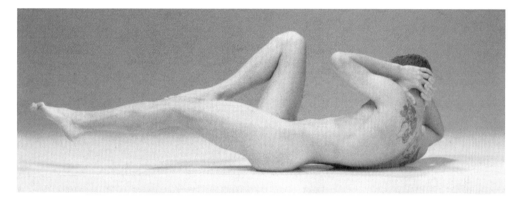

Breathing in slowly, the right elbow compresses toward the left knee, lifting the torso slightly. With a piston-like motion your right leg extends parallel to the floor. Your heel is fully extended with the toes pointing away.

Breathing out slowly, return to your starting position.

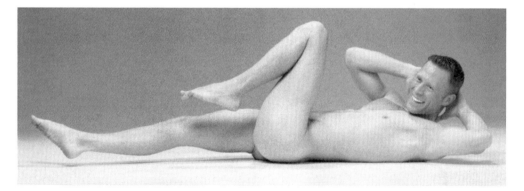

Now the other side: breathing in slowly, your left elbow compresses toward the right knee, lifting the torso slightly. With a piston-like motion your left leg extends parallel to the floor. Your heel is fully extended with the toes pointing away. Repeat twenty times.

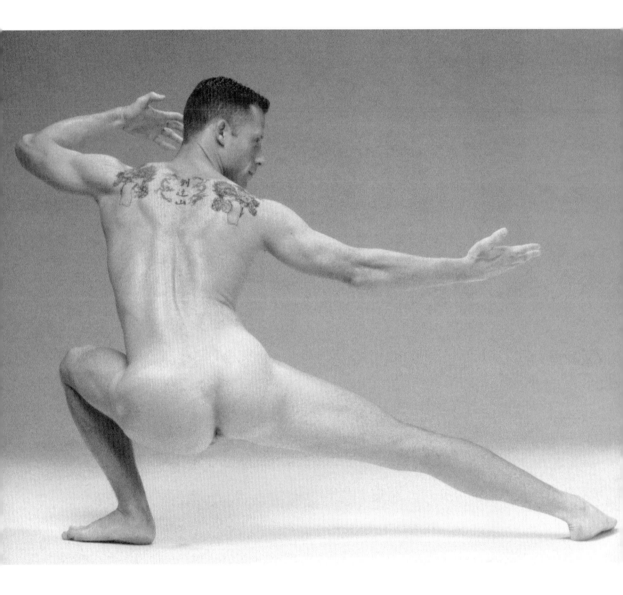

Ins and Outs

Sit with your body tilted back at a forty-five-degree angle. Your legs are lifted up with the knees bent, arms and hands pointing forward for balance. Tighten your abs and glutes for support. Pause and breathe.

Breathe in slowly as you lean farther back, increasing the angle to about sixty degrees. Your legs piston out with a spring-loaded motion. Pause.

Breathing out, slowly return to your starting position. Pause.

Repeat twenty times.

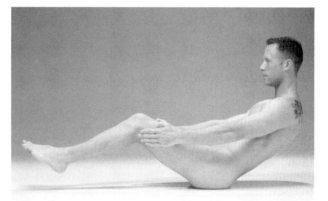

To modify: Rest your hands, palms down, on the deck for balance.

Tip: Perform with slow, fluid movements. Rapid, jerky motion stresses the lower back.

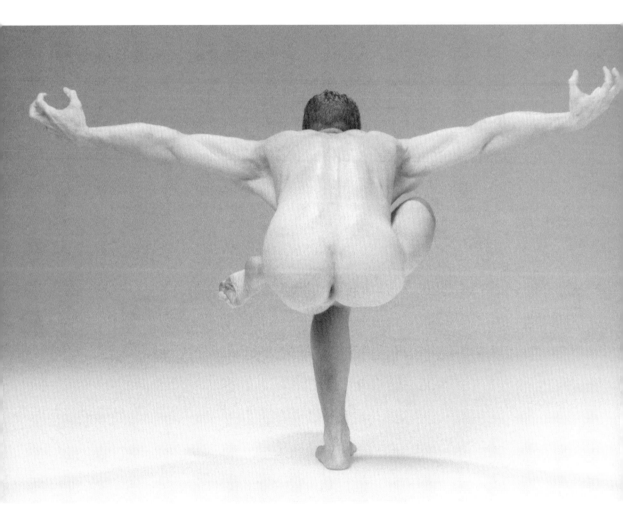

Hindu Squats

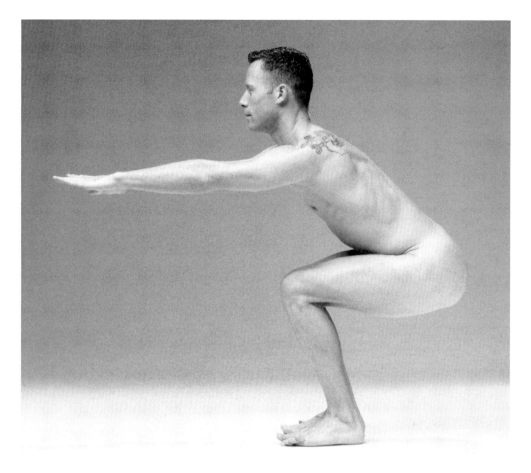

Stand with your feet hip-width apart. Relax your body with your hands resting along the sides of your thighs.

Breathing in slowly, bend your knees and carefully drop your hips toward the floor. As soon as your thighs are parallel to the floor, roll up onto your toes, balancing on the balls of your feet. Be sure to keep your back straight. With a spring-loaded motion raise your arms up to chest height with your hands pointing out in front of you. Pause.

Breathing out slowly, return to standing with your arms resting at your sides. Repeat twenty times.

Tip: Don't lean forward excessively; this places stress on your lower back and knees. As you are dropping into the squat imagine you are sitting into a chair, pointing your hips backward and down.

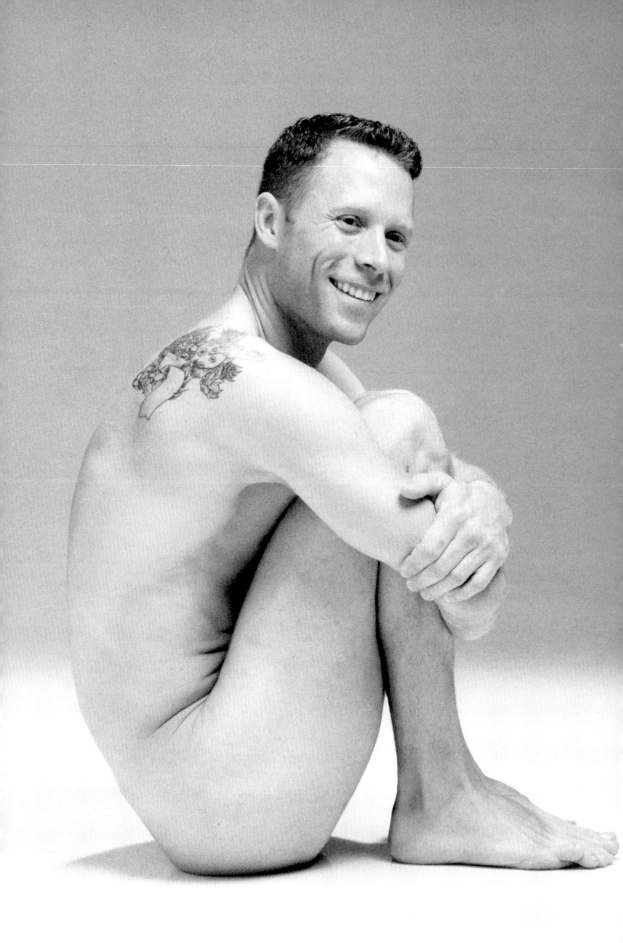

Walking Lunges

Stand with your feet hip-width apart and relax your body, beginning with feet then ankles, legs, knees, hips, pelvis, belly, back, shoulders, jaws, eyes, and scalp. Your hands rest at your sides.

Inhaling slowly, take a giant step forward with your right foot. Carefully lower your left knee toward the floor until it is hovering a few inches above the ground. Your torso is balanced and aligned above your hips with your arms relaxed at your sides. Pause and breathe.

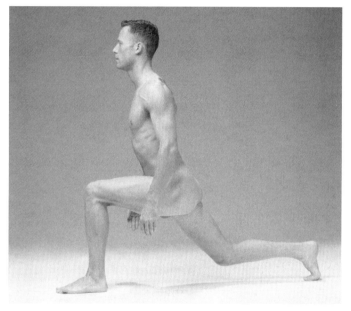

Breathing out, slowly push off with the ball of your left foot, bringing your left foot forward even with your right. Pause and breathe.

Inhaling slowly, take a giant step forward with your left foot. Carefully lower your right knee toward the floor until it is hovering a few inches above the ground. Your torso is balanced and aligned above your hips with your arms relaxed at your sides. Pause and breathe.

Breathing out, slowly push off with the ball of your right foot, bringing your right foot forward even with the left. Pause and breathe.

Repeat alternating legs for twenty strides. (I turn around and lunge to my starting place.)

Tip: Keep the calf of your front foot perpendicular to the floor so as not to put extra stress on your knee.

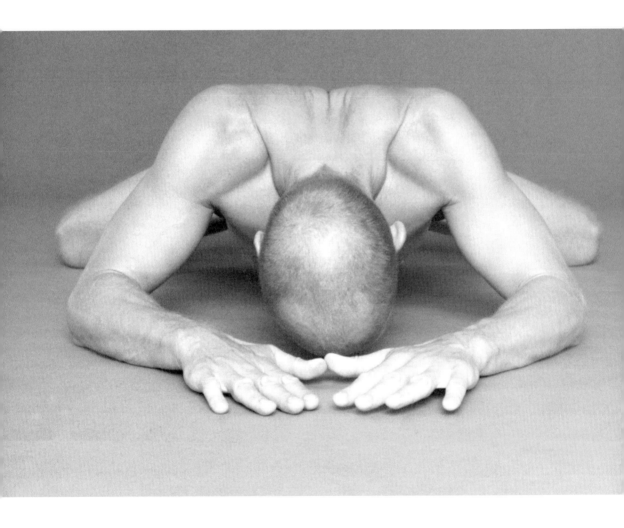

CHAPTER 12

Flexibility

Men are born soft and supple …
plants are born tender and pliant …
Whoever is soft and yielding is a disciple of life.
—*Tao Te Ching,* verse 76 (Mitchell, translation)

Petaluma, California, March 1994: That very first morning at the Lomi School we sat in meditation for an hour. The technique was simple: turn your attention to your body, to the actual sensations of sitting on the mats, your clothing against your skin, your breath moving in and out of your chest. Your body always happens in the now, in the present moment. When you notice yourself thinking, gently bring your attention back to any sensation in your body. Damn! That was simple. I'd been studying meditations for ten years, and no one had explained sitting meditation so plainly.

But simple doesn't always mean easy. For the next hour my uncomfortable body and my restless mind joined forces. I continually reeled my wandering mind back to the sensations of my body—which by then hurt. Sitting on the floor tortured my lazy and out-of-shape body. I ached for the ringing bell to signal the end of the meditation. With very slow movements I stretched my body. That eased the pain. My mind began to focus on my breath, and I finally relaxed. Yet I was grateful when the bell rang.

Next was stretching. Robert Hall introduced us to the "Five Tibetans," which are a series of yoga postures done very quickly. They build strength and flexibility as they move energy throughout the body. "They are the most effective and work the fastest," Robert said. Woven through the Five Tibetans were other Hatha yoga stretches. Robert was sixty years old and amazingly flexible—zipping through the Tibetans with zeal. He cautioned us to "respect the limits of our own bodies and not overdo it. You'll regret it tomorrow."

I continually paused to rest as the class moved through the yoga movements. "Shoulder stand," Robert called out. I watched helplessly as everyone else in the room gracefully rolled up on their shoulders, feet pointing to the ceiling. I couldn't begin to do it. "The Plow," I heard next. Twenty-two sets of feet dropped slowly over their heads toward the floor. I studied the room, half embarrassed and half in awe. I knew I wasn't in Texas anymore.

As I explained above, the exercises known as the Five Tibetans are a series of yoga moves performed quickly in order to create strength and flexibility and allow energy to flow through the body. Mastering these postures, as well as learning how they developed, will illustrate the benefits of making your body more limber.

The Five Tibetans

Every man desires to live long,
But no man wishes to be old.

—Jonathan Swift

The origins of the Five Tibetans are shrouded in romance and legend. As the story goes, a British army colonel learned these exercises from Tibetan monks in an isolated Himalayan monastery. The monks were reported to have found the secrets to a "fountain of youth." The colonel searched for years to find this reclusive sect of monks, and when he reached the monastery, protected by the high mountains and the rough terrain, he was amazed at the health, vitality, and age of the monks. They assured him that the only secrets to their long life were the five yoga exercises, a simple diet, and religious observances.

Returning to Britain, the colonel taught the exercises to Peter Kelder, who published them in a book entitled *Ancient Secrets of the Fountain of Youth* in 1939. Kelder originally called the exercises "the five rites of rejuvenation." Today they are simply known around the world as the Five Tibetans.

The benefits reported by those who practice the Tibetans are increased vitality, flexibility, and mental clarity. There are also many fantastical claims regarding the benefits of these simple exercises. Testimonials included in the introduction to

Kelder's book cite "curing hair loss, memory failure, wrinkles, insomnia, eczema, obesity, arthritis, sinus, pain, and fatigue." Many of these claims are not conclusively documented (or approved by the FDA), but the exercises take a mere ten to twenty minutes a day to do. Their great benefits, compared to the small investment of time and effort, are well worth it.

The Tibetans work on all the vital layers of intelligence. They strengthen the muscles as well as increase flexibility. They enhance breathing and clear the mind. A daily practice requires sheer will. And practitioners report that the exercises are excellent at moving subtle energy through the body.

Whereas a human's gross anatomy refers to the parts we see and use—our limbs, organs, skeleton, muscles—the subtle anatomy deals with the energy centers that connect the body with the higher intelligences. Three distinct examples of the way different parts of the world look at the subtle anatomy include the Hindu belief in the seven chakras; the acupuncture meridian system from the Chinese; and the halo effect that's called the auric field, which is from the Western understanding of energy.

What these three examples have in common is the belief in a spark of divine energy that animates all that is physical about us. This is the level of the soul. It is the level of the spirit. In Eastern theories of medicine, when the subtle energy channels are open and flowing fully, we radiate health.

According to the ancient yoga texts, the seven chakras are lined up in front of the spine, with the first being found at the tip of the tailbone and the seventh at the top of the skull (see Chapter Four). Indian belief teaches that the chakras correspond to the major nerves, glands and tissues throughout the body. Each *chakra*, which means "wheel" or "wheel of spinning light" in Sanskrit, spins on an axis. Increasing the spin of a chakra increases the amount of energy that flows to the associated nerves, glands and organs connected to the chakra. The slower the rate of spin, the less energy flows to the same tissues. With a decreased energy flow the passageways become stagnant or blocked, and the related organs and glands lose their vitality, causing illness and aging.

The Five Tibetans appear to be incredibly successful at increasing the spin of the chakras and thereby the amount of energy that flows through the subtlest layer of consciousness. Practitioners suggest the following conditions to prepare for the Five Tibetans:

- Wear loose clothing.
- Choose a room that lets in fresh air or work outdoors.

- Use a pad of some sort for comfort.

- Consult with a medical doctor or health care practitioner if you are pregnant or have a chronic injury that is painful during exercise.

Each one of the Five Tibetans is a vigorous exercise. They are done quite fast, unlike many of the Hatha yoga movements they resemble, and are repeated twenty-one times, thus becoming an aerobic yoga. Beginners are asked to do seven repetitions (reps) of each exercise. When the student grows stronger, the repetitions increase to fourteen each. Finally, increase each exercise to the full twenty-one reps, the recommended total amount for each exercise (doing more than 21 reps does not seem to increase the benefits of the daily practice).

Synchronizing the breath with the physical movements is the key to these exercises. It is the breath that oxygenates the blood and tissues and clears the mind. I focus on my breathing, allowing the inhale and the exhale of my breath to lead the movements. The effects are quite noticeable.

There is some conflicting advice on how to spin in the first Tibetan. In Kelder's original text he recommends spinning clockwise like the Sufi whirling dervishes. However, this is a contradiction, because the Sufi dervishes spin counterclockwise, and that feels natural to me. So that's how I am explaining the exercise here.

FURTHER READING

Kelder, Peter. *Ancient Secrets of the Fountain of Youth: Book 1*. New York: Doubleday, 1998.

Kilham, Christopher S. *The Five Tibetans*. Rochester, VT: Healing Arts Press, 1994.

Prasad, Rama, and Caroline Robertson. "The Five Tibetans: Easy Energizing Exercises." Available online at www.ayurvedaelements.com/img/five.pdf. Downloaded Sept. 4, 2004.

*Wholesome physical exercise reconstitutes energy,
stemming the aging process, making the body light
and firm, while safeguarding against fatigue
and inducing cheerfulness.*

—Unknown

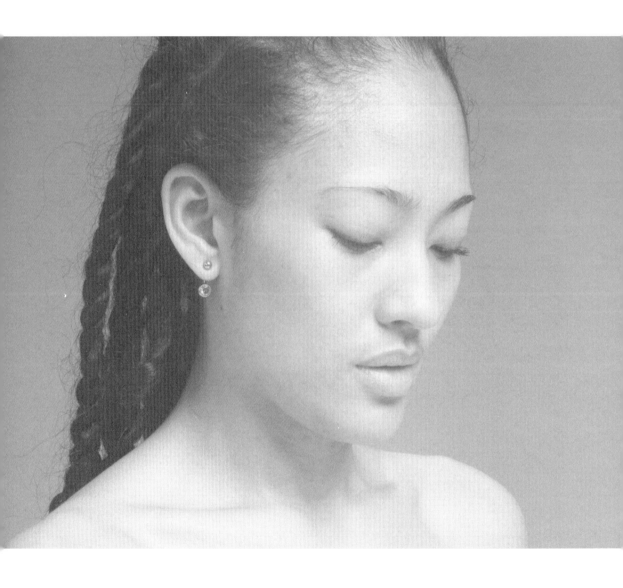

Tibetan One

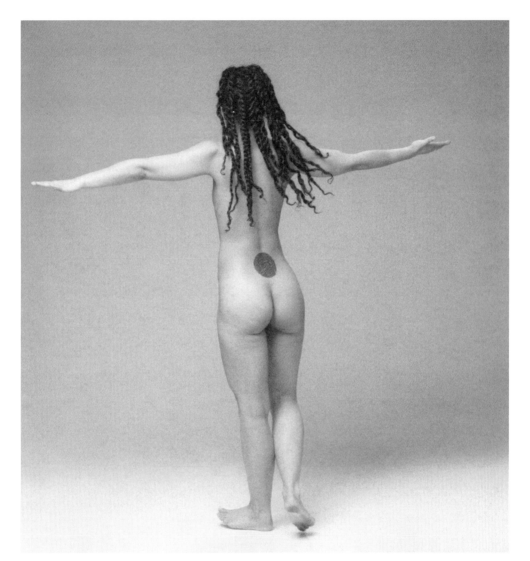

I call this the "dervish," because one spins like Sufi whirling dervishes. Stand with arms outstretched. Find a landmark in the room on which to focus. As you spin past the landmark you can count off the reps. To honor the dervishes, spin counterclockwise, with one palm turned up toward heaven and the other turned down toward the earth.

Spin around twenty-one times.

Tip: You are likely to feel quite dizzy. Holding a finger in front of your eyes focuses your attention and, ideally, keeps you from falling down.

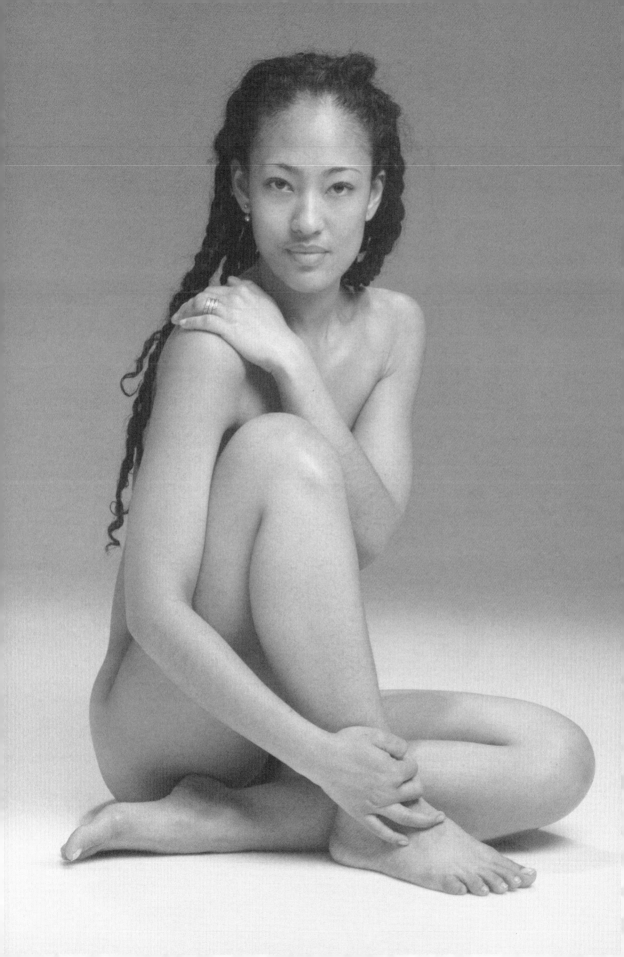

Tibetan Two

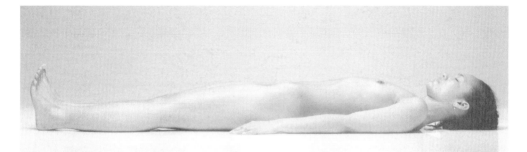

Lie flat on your back.

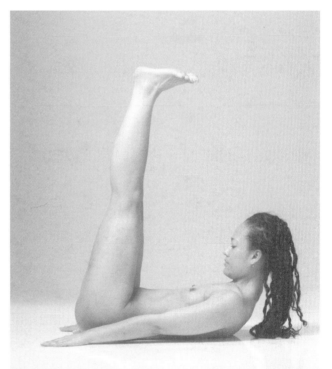

Breathe in deeply as you roll your chin to your chest and lift your legs until they are perpendicular to the floor.

Breathe out as you return to lying flat.

Repeat twenty-one times.

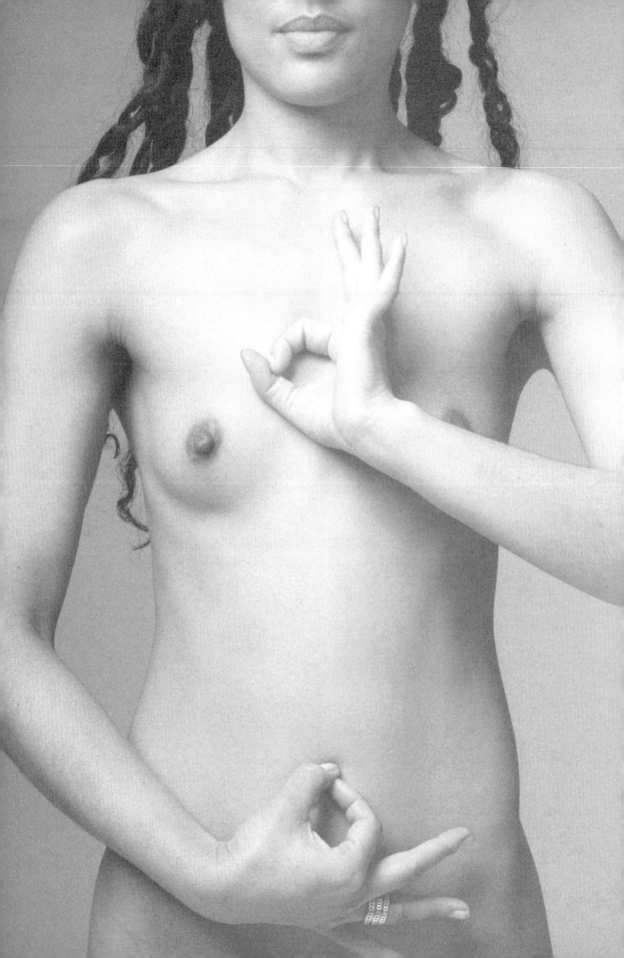

Tibetan Three

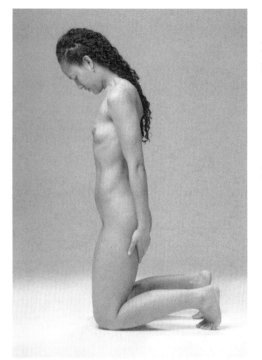

Kneel with your palms gently holding the backs of your thighs.

Breathing in, drop your chin toward your chest.

Breathe out and thrust your chest forward as you lift your chin toward the ceiling.

Repeat twenty-one times.

Tip: I keep my throat strong and the back of my neck soft by pointing my chin to the sky. This gives me a sense of a long throat. This emphasis on "strong throat, soft neck" keeps the vertebrae of my neck from pinching any nerves.

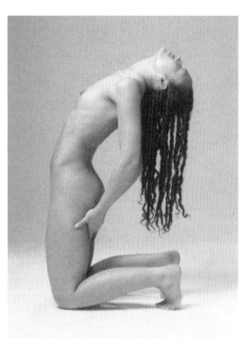

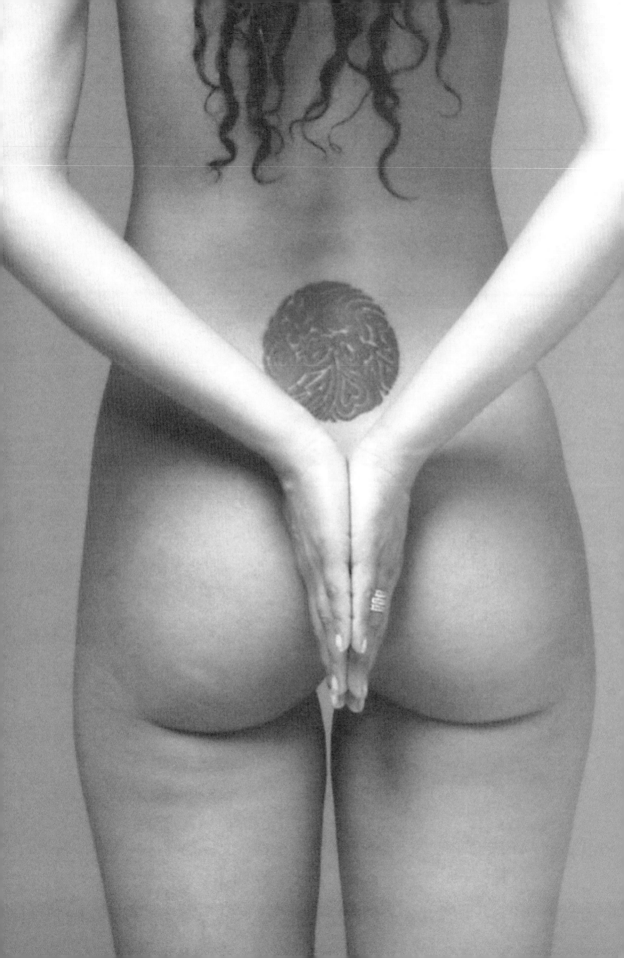

Tibetan Four

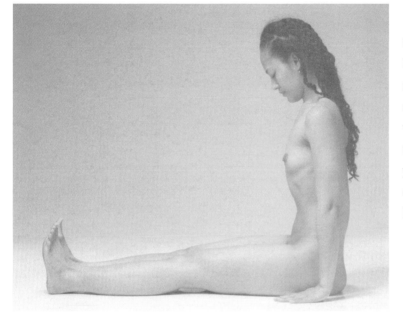

Sit on the floor, back straight and legs out-stretched, with your feet together. Place your hands palm down, by your hips.

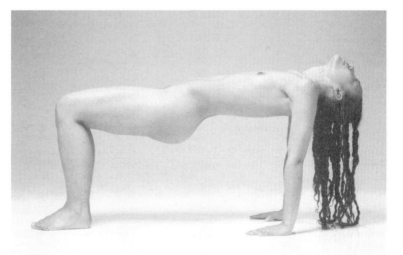

Breathing in, tighten your abdominal muscles and glutes as you lift your hips toward the ceiling. Your chin points toward the sky. Your torso forms a table above the ground.

Breathing out, relax the hips and return to sitting position.

Repeat twenty-one times.

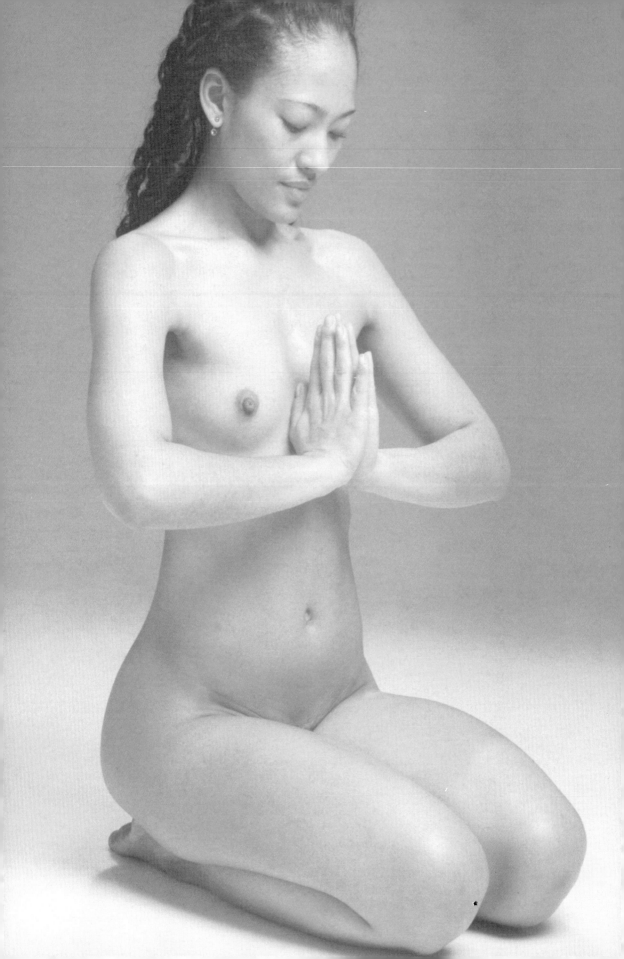

Tibetan Five

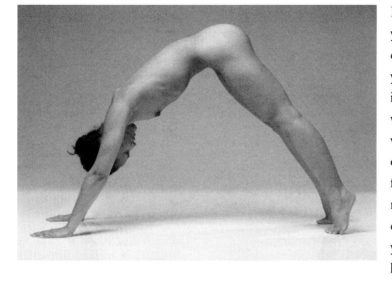

Lie facedown with your hands, palms down, resting by your chest. Lift into a push up, walk your feet forward and roll up on the balls of your feet. Your body makes an upside-down "V." Stretch your arms and legs long.

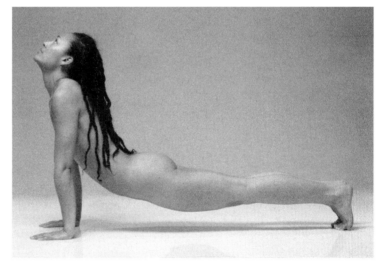

Breathing in, glide your chest toward the floor with your body between your arms. Your legs are parallel along the ground and your chest is thrust forward.

Breathing out, reverse the movement into your beginning position.

Repeat twenty-one times, back and forth.

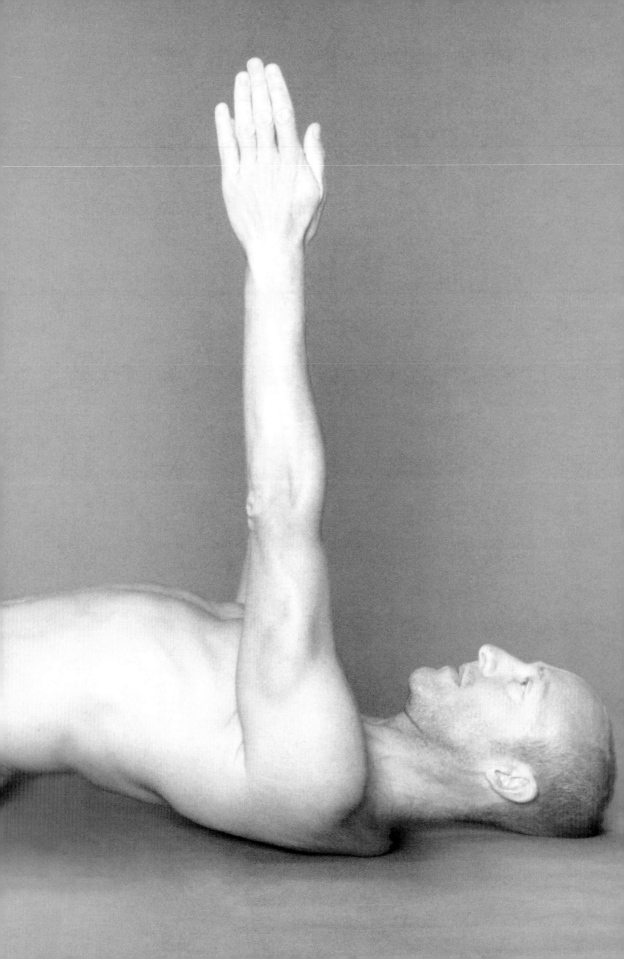

CHAPTER 13

Yoga Down

Everything is in a state of vibration; everything is energy waves. Your body also vibrates at a specific wavelength. You learn to tune to specific wavelengths to get specific energy for strength or power.
—Swami Vishnu-devananda

Houston, Summer 2000: "Downward-facing dog," called out Kay Wescott, my yoga teacher. Like a dog doing a lazy wake-up stretch, she stood on all fours and stretched out her arms and chest, her body a sinuous upside-down "V."

I did my best to follow suit, spreading my fingers wide and pressing my butt into the air. (I couldn't help but chuckle to myself in a moment of cheap humor, then I remembered this was an ancient spiritual tradition.) My spine elongated and I pressed my heels down toward the floor to stretch out my hamstrings. I was breathing harder now and the sweat began to drip from my face and pool between my hands. Breathe, I thought. As one part of my mind calmed with the meditative focus and the exertions of my body, another not-so-quiet voice at the back of my mind whined, "How long can this go on?"

"Crescent moon," called Kay. My mind was momentarily relieved to let go of that down dog. I brought my right foot between my hands into a "runner's lunge" and relaxed my left leg to the floor, pressing my hips forward. My groin muscles stretched easily. I calmly brought my hands to my heart in prayer position—breathe, I remembered. Feeling balanced and with my hands clasped together, I reached toward the ceiling. "Arch those chests forward," urged Kay. I gently curved my back into the beautiful sliver of a crescent moon. (Okay, it's been a while since I've been a sliver of anything, but I could imagine.) I noticed in the mirror that my moon, beautiful as it was, tilted just a little. "Okay yoga monsters, back into down dog," cheered Kay. And so it went through the hour: stretching, pressing, breathing, thrusting, holding, and focusing. Calm mind. Whining mind. Vain mind. Humble mind.

America is abuzz about yoga. The poses known as Sun Salutations are a staple now on American TV. Statistics from *The New York Times* estimate that as many as 12 million Americans do yoga. Forty percent of American health and fitness centers offer Hatha yoga, with more facilities added all the time. A recent search on Amazon. com pulls up more than 1,350 yoga book titles.

Celebrity interest in yoga definitely fuels the hype. In the 1960s, the Beatles sparked interest in yoga by traveling to India to study with the Maharishi Mahesh Yogi. During the 1970s, actors Jeff Bridges, Ruth Buzzi, and Tom Smothers posed for photographs in Bikram Choudhury's book, *Bikram's Beginning Yoga Class.* In the 1980s musician Sting and David Duchovny of "The X-Files" both became devotees, and Ali MacGraw released her own yoga video. Recent converts include Jennifer Aniston and Gwyneth Paltrow.

And of course, in the 1990s, the one-time "Material Girl" herself, Madonna, got serious about her daily yoga practice. Her CD, "Ray of Light," was deeply inspired by her exploration of yoga; she even studied Sanskrit and chanting. And in the film *The Next Best Thing,* Madonna played an Ashtanga yoga teacher. (Ashtanga is an advanced style of yoga requiring more strength and endurance than the better-known Hatha yoga.)

But aside from the hype and the heavy breathing, Westerners find yoga one of the most accessible and useful of the Eastern disciplines. *Yoga* translated from the Sanskrit means "union" or to "yoke together": a discipline, according to Kenneth Davis in his book *Don't Know Much About Mythology,* "designed to link the physical body and mind with the unconscious soul." In India, there are eight schools, or limbs, of the yoga path that attract different personalities and spiritual temperaments, as follows:

- *Raja* ("royal") to control the intellect
- *Hatha* to master the body
- *Kriya* for spiritual action
- *Karma* for selfless action

- *Bhakti* for heartfelt devotion

- *Jnana* to promote knowledge or wisdom

- *Tantra* to enhance truth and non-dual awareness

- *Mantra* for the sacred sounds

- *Kundalini* to understand the subtle energy of the chakras.

Each school has its own teachings and sacred texts, accumulated over the centuries, from which to study.

Over the years, I have seen how stretching complements the massage and bodywork I offer to clients and receive myself. The effects on the muscles and connective tissues are dramatic. I know my own posture has improved, and I feel more graceful as I move through space. Thanks to the yoga *asanas,* which mean "steady pose," I know I'm more flexible.

But flexibility represents much more than just stretching the muscles or connective tissues. Flexibility may sound superficial ("Does it really matter if I can't touch my toes?"), but being limber actually retards aging. An article in a recent *Yoga Journal* explained that:

> *Even if you're active, your body will dehydrate and stiffen with age. By the time you become an adult, your tissues have lost about 15% of their moisture content, becoming less supple and more prone to injury. This normal aging of tissue is distressingly similar to the process that turns animal hides into leather. Unless we stretch, we dry up and tan.*

Good stretching affects three different parts of our bodies: the nerves, the muscle fibers, and the connective tissues. The muscles must be able to fully stretch, to contract, and to rest. These seemingly simple tasks allow us to stand upright, to move, to work, and to play. Returning to full rest after a movement reflects muscle tone or tonus. To achieve tone, muscles rely on the feedback system of our nerves and their own natural elasticity. Accidental injuries, bone fractures, or surgery interfere with the interplay of the nerves and tone of the muscles.

Our muscles develop learned habits. Repeated muscle movements—ranging over a period of time—are the simplest form of body learning. However, very subtle but poor movement habits also affect muscle tone. If a muscle completely relaxes after a movement it has a tonus of zero. If, however, a muscle does not completely relax after its movement, the tonus can climb to 10, 20, 30 or even 40%. Thomas Hanna wrote in his book *Somatics,* "If the tonus is 10%, the muscle will always feel tired and firm. If the tonus is 20%, the muscle will feel tired, very firm and sore. If the tonus is 40%, the muscle will feel tired, hard, and quite painful." Stretching exercises soften muscle tonus, relaxing hard muscles, and allowing them to rest.

The most common connective tissues are our tendons and ligaments. Each muscle has microscopic strands of connective tissue running through it. Every muscle also has an envelope of connective tissue surrounding it called fascia. When you feel like your muscles are all knotted up, it's actually the fascia surrounding the muscles that have gotten stuck together.

The connective tissues are made up of collagen, which strengthens them, and elastin, which gives them elasticity. The "tanning" process is due to dehydration of the connective tissue, resulting in less elastin and more collagen. But flexibility does not rely on the elastin-to-collagen ratio in the connective tissues alone.

Muscle health also depends on its symbiosis with our nerve reflexes. It is our nerve reflexes that control the ability to move and stretch. Over time, however, our nerves contract, establishing a length for each muscle based on how much we move daily. This is called a muscle's "stretch reflex." If we try to move past this stretch reflex point, the nerves revolt and cause a muscle spasm. We feel their pain.

There are several ways to re-educate a muscle's stretch reflex. The first is simply to wait it out. Hatha yoga relies on this traditional method of stretching by encouraging the student to go as far into a stretch as one can safely hold that position. If that pose occurs in concert with concentrated breathing, supported by good strength, the nerve's stretch reflex will exhaust itself. Once this happens, the student ekes out a little more movement until the stretch reflex kicks back in; he waits for relief then repeats the series.

Another way to lengthen a muscle is to bend as fully into a stretch as you safely can, hold it, and breathe for a minute. Then contract the muscle you are trying to stretch for a few seconds to a few minutes. This is called "contract-relax stretching." The muscle contraction suppresses the stretch reflex. As soon as you relax your muscles, immediately push a bit more stretch. The suppression of the reflex is only a split second so move quickly but carefully. Pavel Tsatsouline, the author of *Relax into Stretch,* says studies indicate that contract-relax stretching is "at least 267% more effective than conventional 'wait it out' stretching."

A powerhouse way to lengthen a muscle is to add holding your breath to the contract-relax stretch. Bend as far into the pose as you safely can. Inhale and hold your breath as you contract the muscle you are stretching. I find fifteen to thirty seconds is ample time to override the stretch reflex. Exhale and stretch a little farther. Breathe for a moment, then repeat the combination until your muscles are stretched as far as they will go. Hold that fully stretched pose for a few full breaths.

Flashback to my yoga class: Kay was leading us in the "crow," and the pose challenged even her that morning. "Ohhh," I groaned audibly. The "crow" was an advanced position that I just couldn't seem to master. I slowly bent my knees into a squat and placed my hands on the floor. The idea was to crouch forward, balancing the knees just above the elbows, lift the feet of the floor and support the whole body with the hands. Yes, I agree, theoretically it sounded impossible, but I tried anyway, shifting my weight forward and teetering precariously on my hands and big toes.

In a perfect world I would have lifted my feet in the air and balanced gracefully, gazing serenely into the mirrors ahead. In reality, I huffed and puffed and struggled. Kay encouraged me to "Be patient" and to "Respect the gifts and limits of my body this morning." She also reminded me that I'm a "big crow." My frustration receded, and I vowed to master the pose. In the Chinese calendar, 2000 was the Year of the Dragon, but I vowed to make it the Year of the Crow!

"Are you ready for that *shavasana* (corpse pose)?" Kay teased. "Lie down on your back and do some long body stretches." I lay down and let my feet splay out. I rolled my head from side to side so that it rested naturally. I consciously scanned my body and relaxed: my reward after an intense hour of breathing and stretching. As my body cooled, I felt peaceful, my mind focused and calm, and my emotions riding crisply on the surface of my awareness. My spirit was grateful and soaring. Sure, I was aware of other tightness in my body, yet I was satisfied and pleased with myself. And that is why I continue to practice yoga.

Consciousness seeks our attention to the obvious as well as to the subtle. When we are still, whether sitting quietly or sleeping, our bodies continue to move: our hearts beat, our brains emit waves of energy, and our chests rise and fall as we breathe. Hatha yoga so excellently exemplifies somatic exercise because the regimen focuses on breathing techniques and paying close attention to the subtlest sensations of the body during movement.

When we are attuned to the raw physicality of our bodies, we hone our powers of concentration and relax the mind. A relaxed mind, in turn, is engaged in the present moment, focused on the "now." Our bodies live in the present, never the past nor the future. By paying attention to the bare bones of a simple movement, we can then expand that level of concentration to become acutely aware of our bodies, our emotions, our thoughts and beliefs, and our behaviors—the truths of our lives. After all, life is movement.

FURTHER READING

Budilovsky, Joan, and Eve Adamson. *The Complete Idiot's Guide to Yoga*. New York: Alpha Books, 1998.

Choudhury, Bikram, and Bonnie Jones Reynolds. *Bikram's Beginning Yoga Class*. New York: Tarcher/Putnam Books, 1978.

Davis, Kenneth C. *Don't Know Much About Mythology*. New York: HarperCollins, 2005.

Hanna, Thomas. *Somatics*. Reading, MA: Addison-Wesley Publishing, 1988.

Tsatsouline, Pavel. *Relax into Stretch*. St. Paul, MN: Dragon Door Publishing, 2001.

Don't go outside your house to see flowers.
My friend, don't bother with that excursion.
Inside your body there are flowers.
One flower has a thousand petals.
That will do for a place to sit.
Sitting there you will have a glimpse of beauty
Inside the body and out of it,
Before gardens and after gardens.

—Kabir

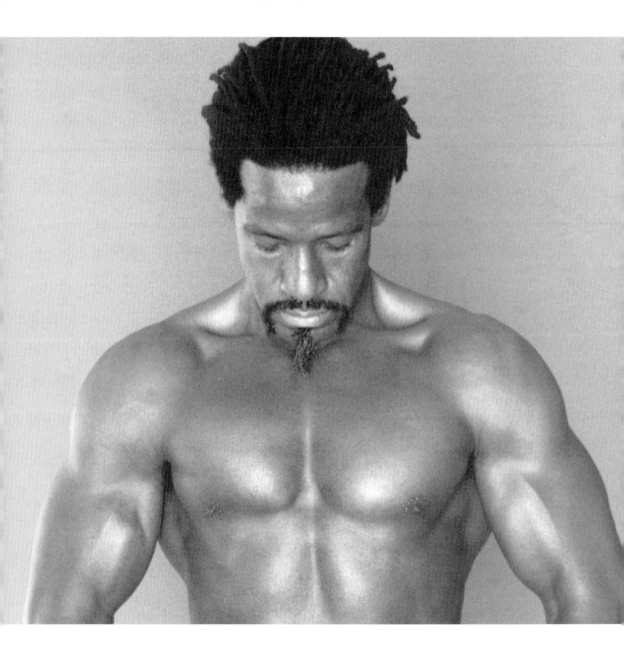

CHAPTER 14

The Rishikesh Series

Yoga is 99% practice and 1% knowledge.
—Sri Krishna Pattabhi Jois

Houston, Late Spring 1993: The room was just large enough for the two of us to lie still, like corpses, on the floor. Black bookshelves holding a gargantuan library towered over us. Champa incense smoldered on the desk as James clanged pots and pans in the kitchen downstairs; my mouth watered with the aroma of dinner. Roy's voice, sounding next to me, brought me back from my calm. "Wiggle your toes and stretch your body. Come back to the room when you're ready." I had just had my first private yoga session.

Roy Oakes was a man of contrasts. I had met him in the early 1980s; at that time Roy was a computer whiz kid and a major-league party boy. My own party days were winding down, but Roy, like most of the boys in Montrose, was still riding high. I had offered to co-host the Grey Party, one of Houston's biggest parties and AIDS fund-raisers. Roy, James Stevenson, and their friend Stella hosted a planning meeting for the event at their posh high-rise apartment. My curiosity was piqued that night by the copy of the *Tao Te Ching* carefully placed on the coffee table. Following the meeting, we struck up a conversation about the book of Chinese wisdom and became friends.

Rich's, the bar where I worked, was the swinging disco in those days. The three-some, as Roy, James, and Stella were called, along with the "twinage"—Lynn and Julia, who are identical twins—started coming to the bar. That was quite a feat as my bar was situated at the top of a steep concrete stairwell, and Stella was permanently in a wheelchair. That didn't stop Roy and James. They joyfully pulled her backward up the stairs, Stella waving all the while to the boys climbing behind her. Once at the top of the stairs, she sure could twirl in that wheelchair. We had fun.

Roy and James soon left for New York, where Roy worked for the investment house Goldman Sachs and James for the designer Norma Kamali. After a few years of the fabulous fast life, rising debt, and weakening immune systems, they came home to Houston. They were determined to beat AIDS and the HIV virus using natural and alternative therapies. That meant low-stress (and low-paying) jobs. Roy went to work at A Moveable Feast, a health-food store and restaurant, and James did display windows at Neiman Marcus. Thus I learned of Roy's other life.

As a young man fresh out of high school Roy lived in Bremen, Germany. While there he answered an ad in the local paper for an ongoing yoga class that taught the Rishikesh series, named for the meditation ashram in Rishikesh, India. Over the year, members of the class reported much-improved health and flexibility and described dramatic changes, for the better, in their personal lives. The class attributed these benefits to their ongoing yoga practice.

Roy said the ten poses he learned really worked for him. I was intrigued. Roy had spent years living at an ashram in Denton, Texas, where he practiced meditation and yoga and experimented with some LSD and magic mushrooms (it was the 1970s). When AIDS came knocking Roy had a full spiritual life to fall back on. He and James designed new and healthy lifestyles for themselves. Roy rekindled a nightly yoga and meditation program.

That first lesson in Roy's study was an eye-opener. Doing yoga hurt me, or, I should say, stretching my body hurt me. My pathologically lazy life had repaid me with amazingly tight muscles and stiff joints. My body was rigid. I decided then and there that I didn't have the time or the interest for yoga, and I did not try it again until my sojourn at the Lomi School.

But as my appreciation for yoga has grown over the years, I have returned, again and again, to the Rishikesh series Roy taught me. Looking for a good quote on yoga, I picked up *The Sivananda Companion to Yoga,* and as I thumbed through the pages I recognized most of the poses. Then I saw the word "Rishikesh"! Roy's ten poses were abbreviated from the yoga taught by the Sivananda ashrams, located from Rishikesh, to London, to San Francisco. I was pleased to see that most of the additions I had made to the original series of ten were found in the Sivinanda warm-up or extended series.

"How often do we need to stretch?" is a good question with a lot of different expert answers. "Nearly every day" is the best answer. At the very least stretch one day for every day you exercise: lift weights, run, swim, play volleyball, or participate in any sport. Sport activities tend to shorten the muscles during play. If the muscles are not stretched to counterbalance the shortening they habitually tighten, causing pain and possible injury.

A recent article on preventing sports injuries in *The New York Times* quoted Dr. Gloria Beim, an orthopedic surgeon in Crested Butte, Colorado. She is the team doctor for the U.S. track cycling team. Beim recommended aerobic movement to warm up the muscles followed by aggressive stretching before any sports activity. She also said, "I tell my patients, 'Stretching right before you exercise three times a week isn't going to do it. You need to stretch every day to get its benefit.'"

Roy taught me to begin each yoga session with the Sun Salutation. This is a famous series of exercises that flow through a dozen steps and are performed a dozen times. This flow of exercises, or *Vinyasa,* warms up the body so that it is limber and prepared for the formal Rishikesh poses.

Over time I substituted the Five Tibetans for the Sun Salutations. I also have included the written instructions for some all-purpose light stretches to warm and loosen the body before one attempts the stronger Rishikesh poses—do what works for you.

Warm-up Stretches

The following are some simple exercises to wake up and limber the body. All of these movements work more effectively in combination with the traditional Hatha yoga breath for stretching: Ujjayi (prohounced oo-JAH-ya). I call it the Darth Vader breath.

- Keeping your lips closed inhale slowly through your nose. Close your glottis, which is just above your vocal chords; this gives your breath that Darth Vader sound. Breathe fully into your belly.

- Exhale slowly through your nose with your lips closed. You're now ready for the warm-ups.

Hip Spirals

- Stand with your feet hip-width apart. Relax your body beginning with feet, then ankles, legs, hips, pelvis, belly, shoulders, jaws, eyes, and scalp.

- Breathing normally, slowly begin to draw a small circle with your tailbone. Notice the sensations through your whole body with this simple movement. Gradually allow your tailbone to spiral outward. The movement of your hips becomes more exaggerated with each spiral, until your hands dip a little toward the floor with each pass.

- Stop wherever you are. Feel the unusualness of this exaggerated pose. Reverse the spiral, slowly moving your way back to your center, then stop and notice the sensations in your body.

- One repetition in each direction.

Neck Rolls

- Stand with your feet hip-width apart. Relax. Breathing normally, slowly drop your chin to your chest. Slowly roll your chin to your left collarbone.

- Continue rolling your head so that your left ear drops toward your left shoulder. Feel the stretch in the right side of your neck. Slowly let your head roll to your back with your chin pointing up. Let your head roll to the right so that the right ear drops toward the right shoulder. The chin rolls toward the right collarbone and back to the chest.

- Do two more full neck rolls in this direction.

- Repeat entire sequence rolling head to the right three full times.

Tip: Pointing your chin upward toward the sky keeps the weight of your head from pinching the nerves between your vertebrae.

Spinal Rolls

- Stand with your feet hip-width apart. Relax. Soften your knees and slowly drop your chin to your chest. Allow the weight of your head to draw you toward the ground. Your back curls forward one vertebra at a time until you are gently hanging from your hips.

- Take a deep breath. If you need to, place the heels of your hands on your knees for support. Slowly reverse this movement, restacking the vertebrae one at a time until you are standing upright, then stop and notice the sensations in your body.

- Repeat two more times.

Tip: If you feel several vertebrae locked together by tension, pause and breathe deeply into those vertebrae.

Windmills

- Stand with your legs spread apart by about double your hip-width with your feet facing straight ahead. Relax. Place your palms together in the prayer position and stretch your arms above your head.

- Breathing slowly, turning your chest over your right thigh and slowly lower your torso so that your palms reach your right foot. Soften your knees if your need to. Slowly swing your palms to your left foot with your chest stretching over your left thigh. Slowly raise your torso back up to a standing position with your palms reaching above you.

- Continue your slow swing back down to your right foot, around to your left foot and back to standing. Do three full rotations to the right.

- Pause. Notice your breath and feel your body. Notice the myriad sensations as you stand.

- Repeat three windmills swinging to the left.

Squats

- Stand with your feet hip-width apart. Relax. Soften your knees and slowly drop your chin to your chest. Allow the weight of your head to draw you toward the ground. Your back curls forward one vertebra at a time until you are gently hanging from your hips.

- Slowly bend your knees and lower your hips toward the floor until you are in a full squat. Pause. Gently drape both hands behind your neck (caution: do not pull) and let gravity gently stretch the extra weight forward. This is an excellent stretch for the lower back.

- Place both palms on your knees. Turn your attention to your sitz bone (the pelvic bone that you actually sit on). Slowly lift your sitz bone up until your legs are straight and you are bent at the waist. Restacking the vertebrae one at a time, slowly raise your torso to standing. Take a deep breath and notice the sensations in your body.

- One full repetition.

Cossack Squats

- Stand with your legs spread wide, your feet facing straight ahead. Relax. Soften your knees and slowly drop your chin to your chest. Allow the weight of your head to draw you toward the ground. Your back curls forward one vertebra at a time until you are gently hanging from your hips.

- Place both palms on the floor. Bend your right knee into a squat. As you do your left leg straightens and rolls so that your left toes point toward the ceiling. With practice your right heel will eventually rest flat on the floor. You should feel the inner thigh of your left leg stretching. Breathe and relax into the stretch.

- Shift your weight to your hands and straighten your right leg so that both legs are straight and you are bent over at the waist. Breathe and relax.

- Bend your left knee into a squat. As you do, your right leg will straighten and roll so that your right toes point toward the ceiling. With practice your left heel will eventually rest flat on the floor. You should feel the inner thigh of your right leg stretching. Breathe and relax into the stretch.

- Shift your weight to your hands and straighten your left leg so that both legs are standing and you are bent over at the waist. Breathe and relax.

- Repeat stretch on both sides two more times.

Crescent Moon

- Stand with your feet hip-width apart. Relax. Soften your knees and slowly drop your chin to your chest. Allow the weight of your head to draw you toward the ground. Allow your back to curl forward one vertebra at a time until you are gently hanging from your hips. Place both hands on the floor.

- Step back with your right leg, which brings you into a lunge position. Rest your right knee and the top of your right foot on the floor. Stabilize yourself and bring your hands to prayer position. Thrust your chest forward. Stretch your hands up toward the ceiling and back behind you. Your hands, arms, torso and right leg form a beautiful crescent arch.

- Bring your hands back to the floor on each side of your left foot. Lift your hips and return to standing.

- Repeat on the left side.

Hamstring Stretch

- Lie flat on your back with your legs straight and feet together. Lift your right leg, keeping it straight as far as you are comfortable. You may use your hands to massage and gently stretch the back of the thigh. Or you may use a strap to hook around the sole of the foot to gently stretch your leg. With practice you will stretch your leg so that you form a ninety-degree angle with your extended leg and the rest of your body. Keep your left toes pointing toward the sky.

- Repeat with your left leg.

FURTHER READING

Lidell, Lucy with Narayani and Giris Rabinovitch. *The Sivananda Companion to Yoga: A Complete Guide to the Physical Postures, Breathing Exercises, Diet, Relaxation, and Meditation Techniques of Yoga.* London, England: Gaia Books, 1983.

Prasad, Rama, and Caroline Robertson. "The Five Tibetans: Easy Energizing Exercises." Available online at www.ayurvedaelements.com/img/five.pdf. Downloaded Sept. 4, 2004.

Visit www.BodyBrillianceBook.com to download your free written copy of these exercises.

First of all the twinkling stars vibrated,
but remained motionless in space,
then all the celestial globes were united into one
series of movements.
… Firmament and planets both disappeared,
but the mighty breath which gives life to all things
and in which all is bound up remained.

—Vincent Van Gogh

Big Al's Rishikesh Series
(with a Twist)

Now that you've warmed up, you are ready to try the Rishikesh Series of poses, adapted by me, as illustrated on the following pages:

- The Triangle: Trikonasana

- The Tree: Vrikshasana

- The Camel: Ustrasana

- Shoulder Stand: Sarvangasana

- The Plow: Halasana

- The Fish: Matsynasana

- Standing Head to Knee: Uttanasana

- The Cobra: Bhujangasana

- The Locust: Salabhasana

- The Bow: Dhanurasana

- Headstand: Shirshasana

- Child's Pose: Mudhasana

- Spinal Twist

- Corpse Pose: Shavasana

Visit www.BodyBrillianceBook.com to download your free written copy of these exercises.

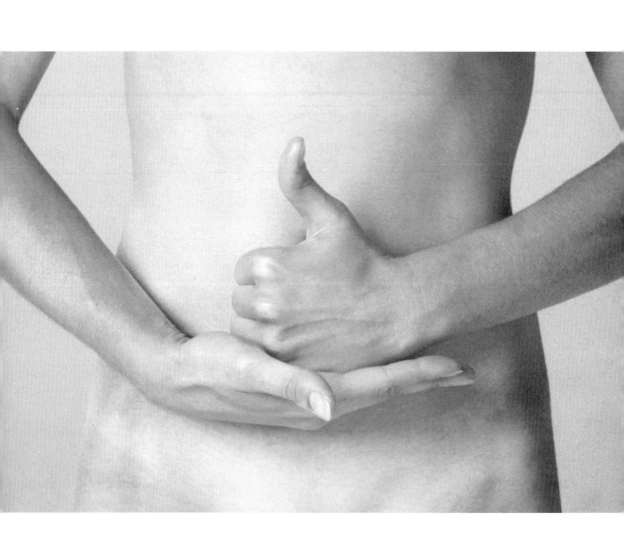

The Triangle

Trikonasana

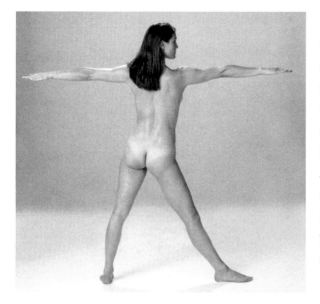

Stand with your feet widely spread. Lift your arms up. Turn your head to look over your right arm. Extend your torso rightward, keeping a straight line with both of your arms. As you bend at the waist reach for your right foot. Soften your right knee if you need to. Place your right hand on your calf, ankle, or the floor.

Turn your chest so that it faces (shines) forward. Both your shoulders are aligned with your right thigh. Your left arm is reaching toward the ceiling.

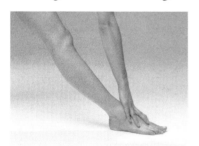

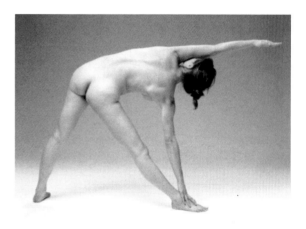

Turn your head and focus your eyes on your left thumb. Relax into the stretch. Now slowly drop your left arm level with your torso. Use the ujjayi (Darth Vader) for ten breaths.

As you are ready raise your left arm back toward the sky. Imagine that a giant hand reaches down and grabs you by your left wrist and pulls you back to standing.

Repeat on your left side.

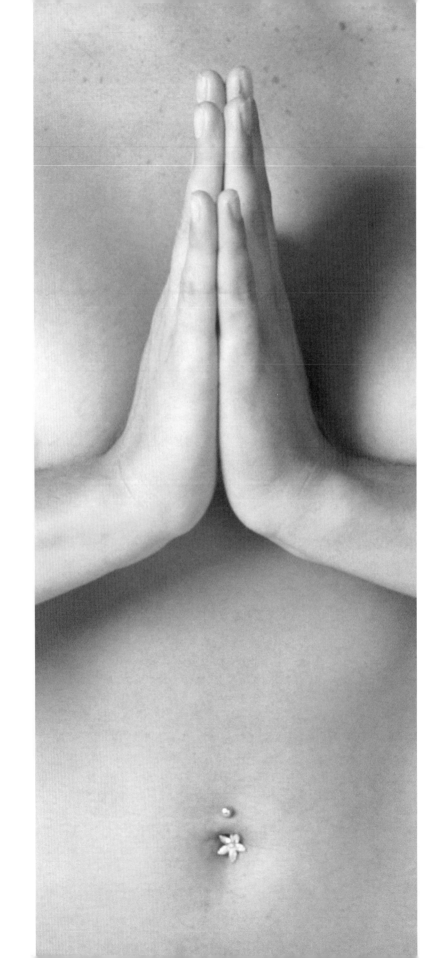

The Tree

Vrikshasana

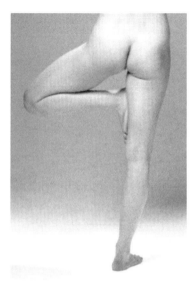

Stand with your feet together, your arms relaxed at your sides.

Bring your left foot to your right calf, knee, or inner thigh.

Tip: Keep both your hips even and facing fully forward.

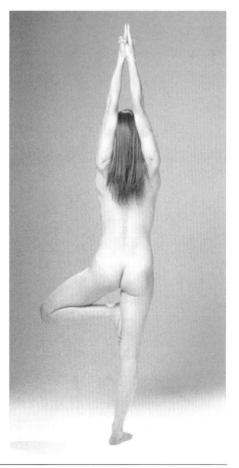

Place both palms together in front of your heart in prayer position.

When you feel steady stretch your arms above your head. Ujjayi breathe and relax for ten breaths.

Return to standing.

Repeat on left side, one time each.

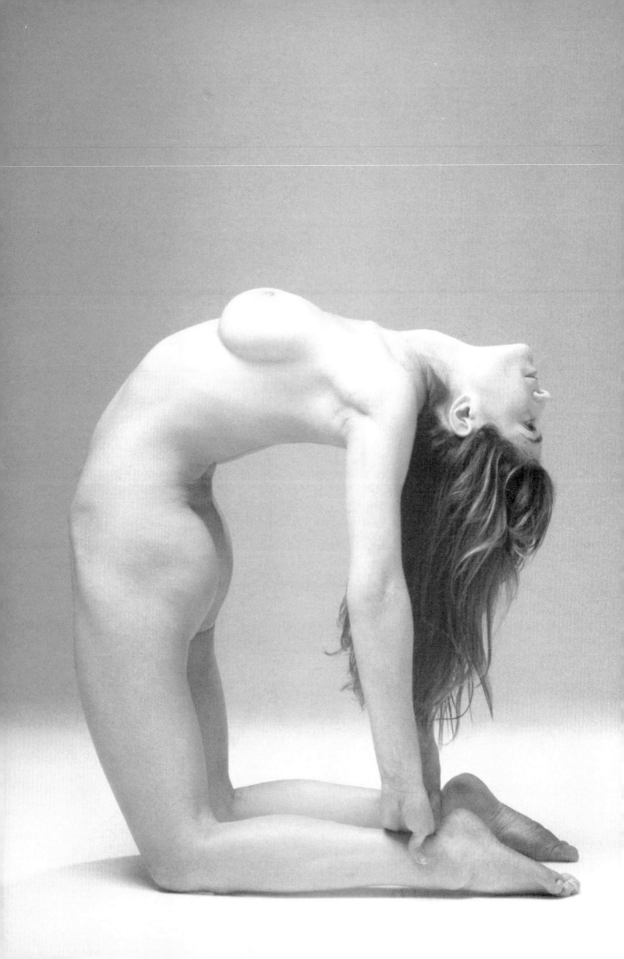

The Camel

Ustrasana

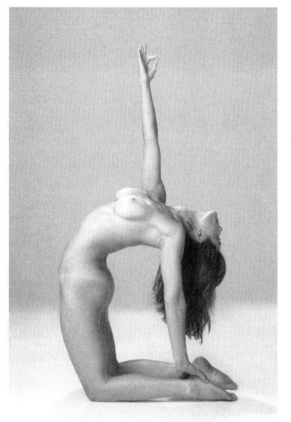

Kneel with your legs and feet slightly apart. Rest your palms on your thighs.

With your left hand slowly grasp your left ankle behind you. Reach your right hand toward the sky. Breathe and relax.

Return to kneeling with your palms resting on your thighs.

Carefully reach back and grasp both ankles. Lift your chest toward the sky. Ujjayi breathe and relax for ten breaths.

Return to kneeling.

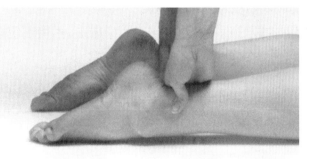

Tip: As you lean back, point the top of your head to the wall behind you. This keeps you from pinching the nerves in your neck.

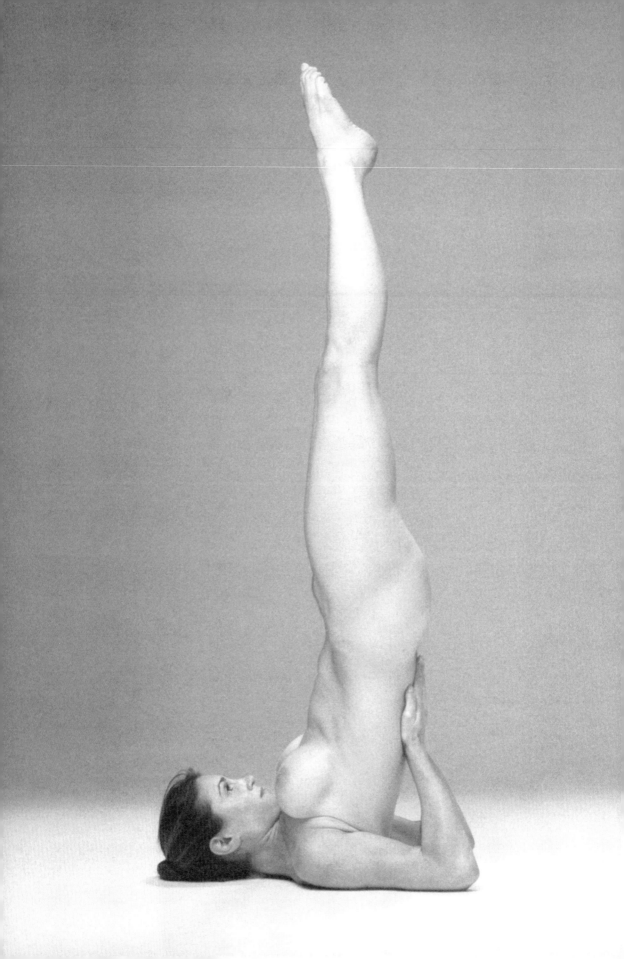

Shoulder Stand

Sarvangasana

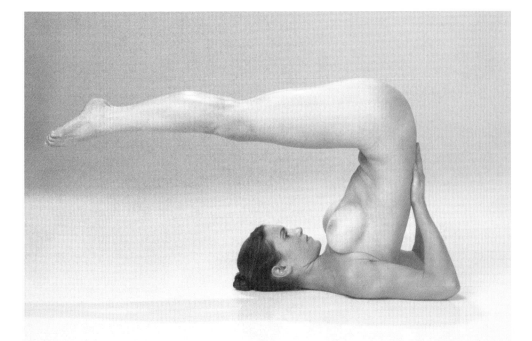

Lie flat on your back with your hands resting at your sides. Keeping your legs straight, slowly lift them up and over your head until your legs are parallel to the floor. Point your toes, and by contracting your abdominal muscles, lift your legs and torso straight up toward the sky. Breathe!

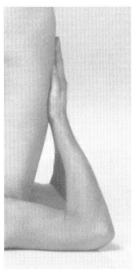

Bring your hands to the middle of your back with your fingers resting along your spine. With careful attention stretch your ears away from your shoulders by pressing your chin into your throat. Ujjayi breathe and hold the pose for ten breaths.

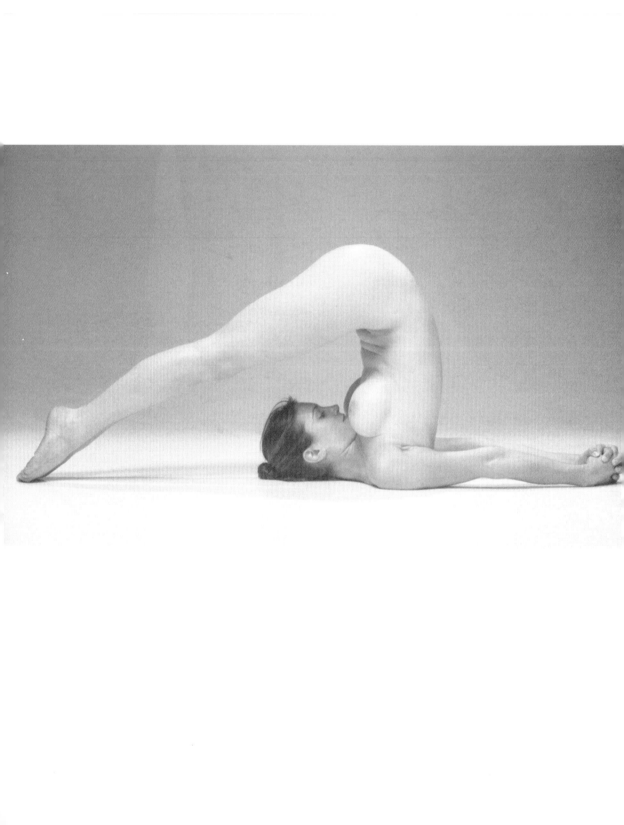

The Plow

Halasana

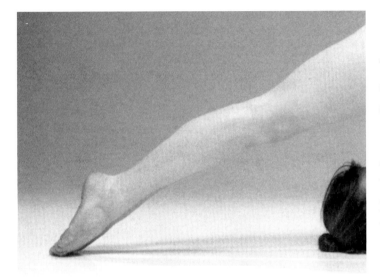

This position is a continuation of the shoulder stand.

Slowly drop your feet to the floor above your head. Keep your toes pointed.

Relax your arms, interlace your fingers, and press your hands away from your back until your arms are straight out on the floor.

Ujjayi breathe and relax for ten breaths.

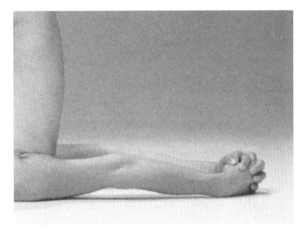

To unfold your body, begin by relaxing your hands and pressing them flat to the floor. Tighten your abdominal muscles and slowly uncurl your body one vertebra at a time. Keep the legs strong and straight until your heels return to the floor.

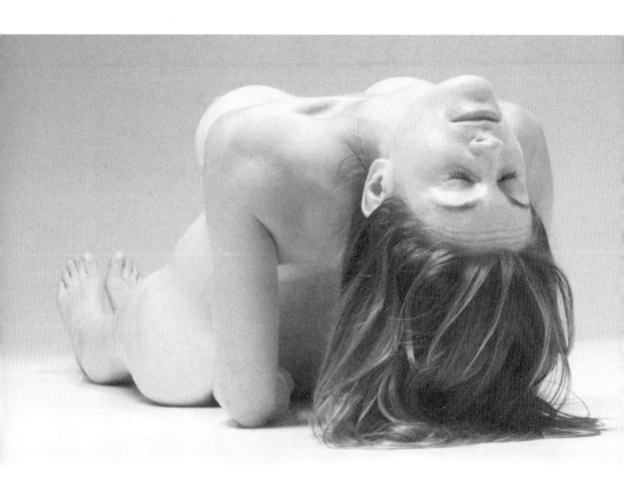

The Fish

Matsynasana

This fish pose stretches open the chest and throat. It is a traditional counter pose to the shoulder stand and the plow.

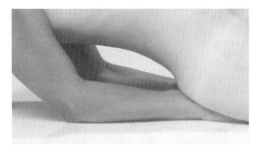

Lie on your back and place your hands, palms down, under your hips.

Slowly press your arms into the floor, arch your back as you gently roll the top of your head to the floor. Ujjayi breathe and relax for five breaths.

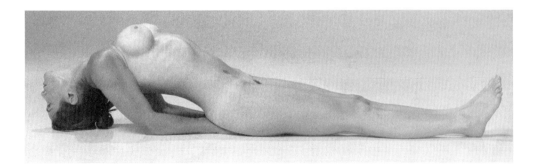

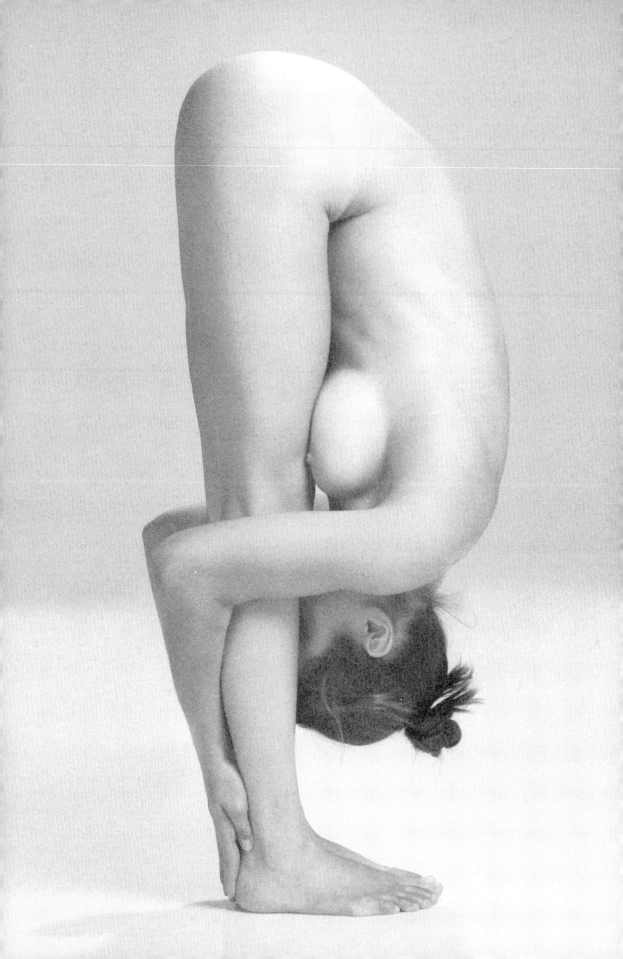

Standing Head-to-Knee

Uttanasana

Be sure your legs are warmed up and relaxed for this one.

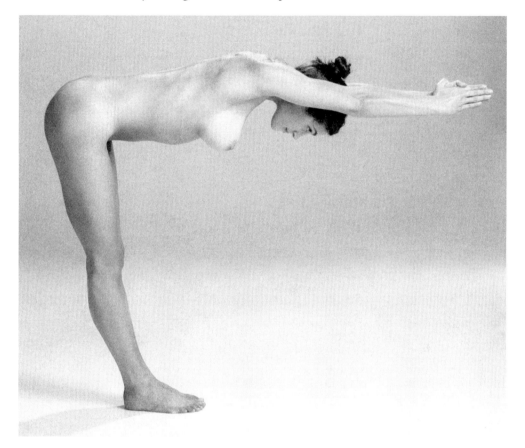

Stand relaxed with your palms together and your hands straight up above your head. Slowly bend your body at the hips while your upper body remains straight and strong. When you are halfway down, your body will make a lovely ninety-degree angle.

Continue folding until your forehead rests against your knees. Wrap your arms gently around your calves and relax them. Ujjayi breathe and relax for ten breaths.

To unfold your body, slowly reverse your movements until you are standing.

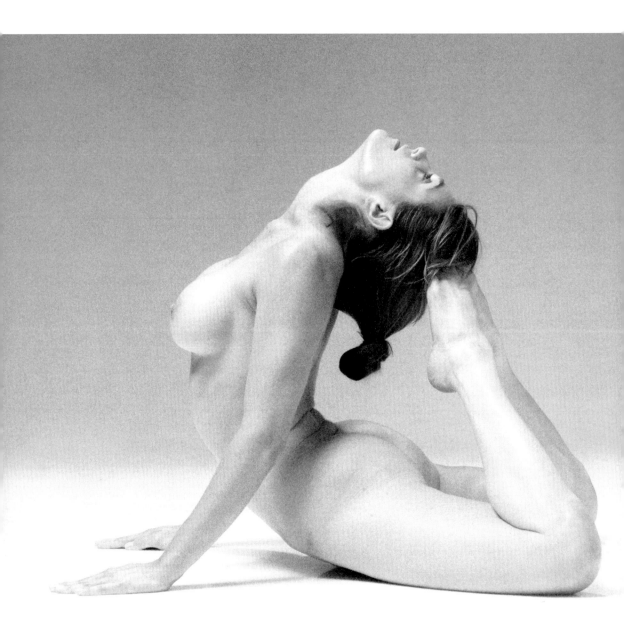

The Cobra

Bhujangasana

This pose lengthens and strengthens your chest and upper back.

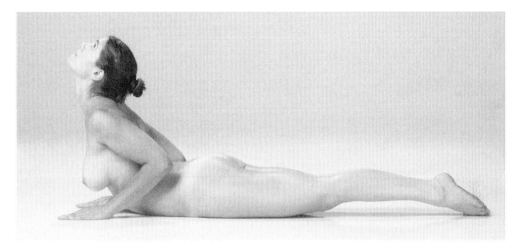

Lie facedown with your palms resting on the floor near your shoulders. Your feet and legs are together. They remain relaxed yet strong.

With a deep breath lift your head by slowly pressing your nose forward and then up. Arch your back until you are looking at the sky.

Ujjayi breathe and relax for ten breaths.

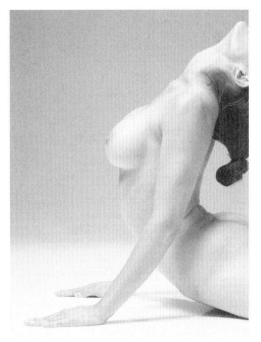

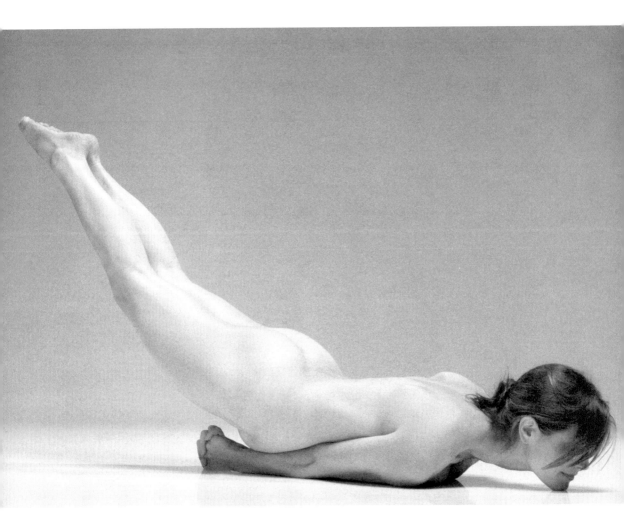

The Locust

Salabhasana

This pose stretches and strengthens the lower back.

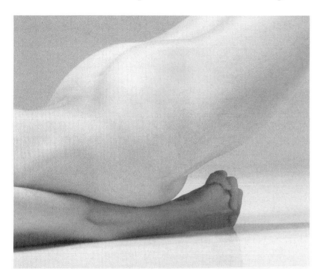

Lie facedown. Bring your fore-arms and hands together under your torso, interlacing your fingers.

The backs of your thumbs rest on the ground.

Start by keeping one leg relaxed and yet strong on the floor. Lift your other leg into the air, pointing your toes up and back. Breathe and hold.

Now switch legs and alternate three times.

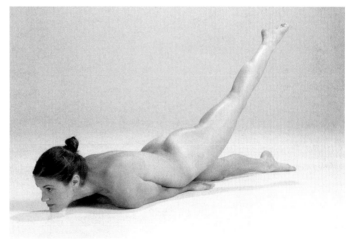

Then lift both legs and hold. Focus on the low back muscles. Take a deep breath. Keeping both legs together lift them up into the air. Ujjayi breathe and relax for ten breaths.

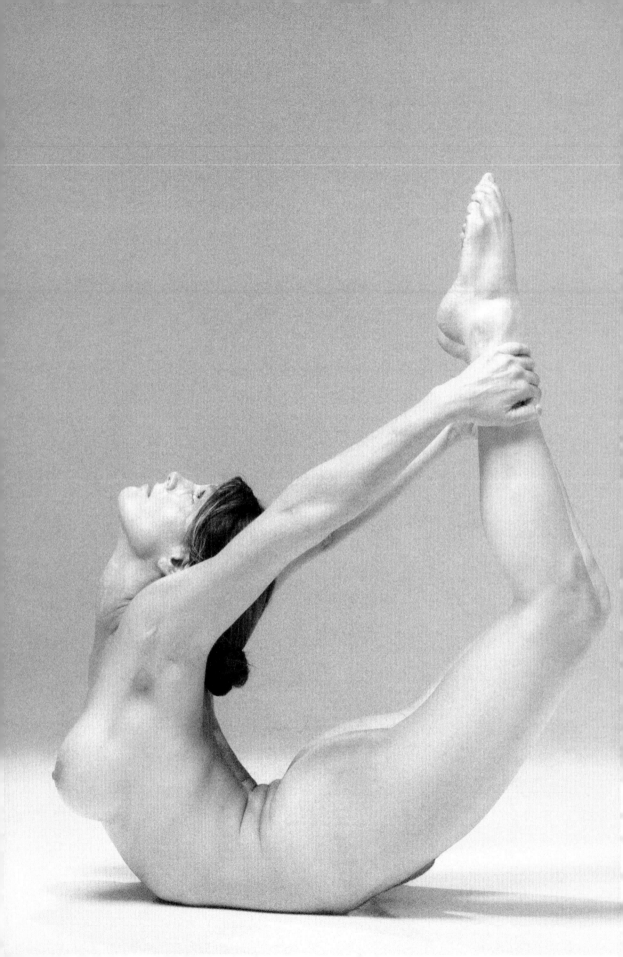

The Bow

Dhanurasana

This pose strengthens the back and stretches the front of the body.

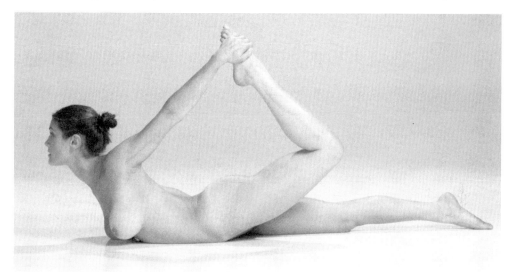

Lie face down. Slowly reach back with your left hand and grasp your left foot, lifting your torso and left thigh off the mat. Hold for three breaths. Return to the resting position.

Slowly reach back with your right hand and grasp your right ankle, lifting your torso and right thigh off the mat. Hold for three breaths. Return to your resting position.

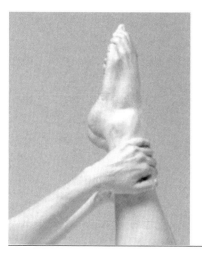

Grasp both your ankles with your hands and lift your feet toward the sky. Ujjayi breathe and relax into the pose for ten breaths.

With a deep breath lower your body back to the mat and release your ankles.

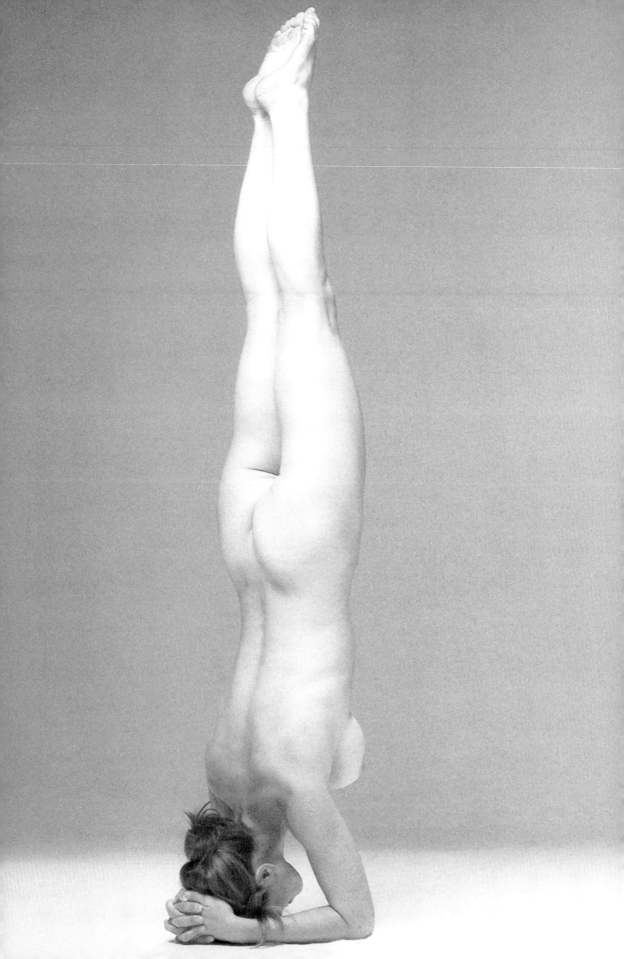

Headstand

Shirshasana

This inversion is the mother of all yoga poses. A good soft surface helps. Beginners may practice this pose against a wall until they feel ready to balance without support.

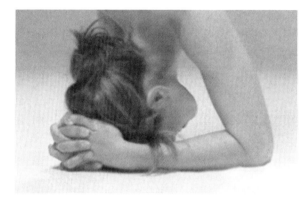

Kneeling, interlace your fingers and place your elbows and forearms on the floor. Your interlocked palms create a tripod with your elbows. Place the top of your head on the ground so that the back of your head rests in the palms of your hands.

Lift your hips up toward the sky, stretching out the back of your legs. Slowly walk your feet toward your head.

Tighten your abdominal muscles and slowly lift your knees toward your thighs. Pause, breathe, and lift your feet to the sky. Focus on keeping your balance as your feet press up. Ujjayi breathe and relax for ten breaths.

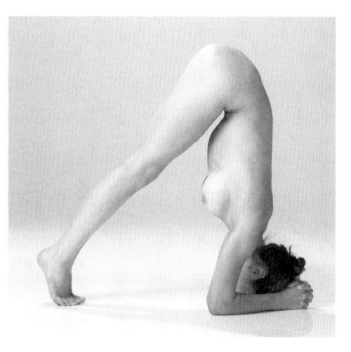

To release, tighten your abs and slowly lower first one straight leg and then the other to the floor.

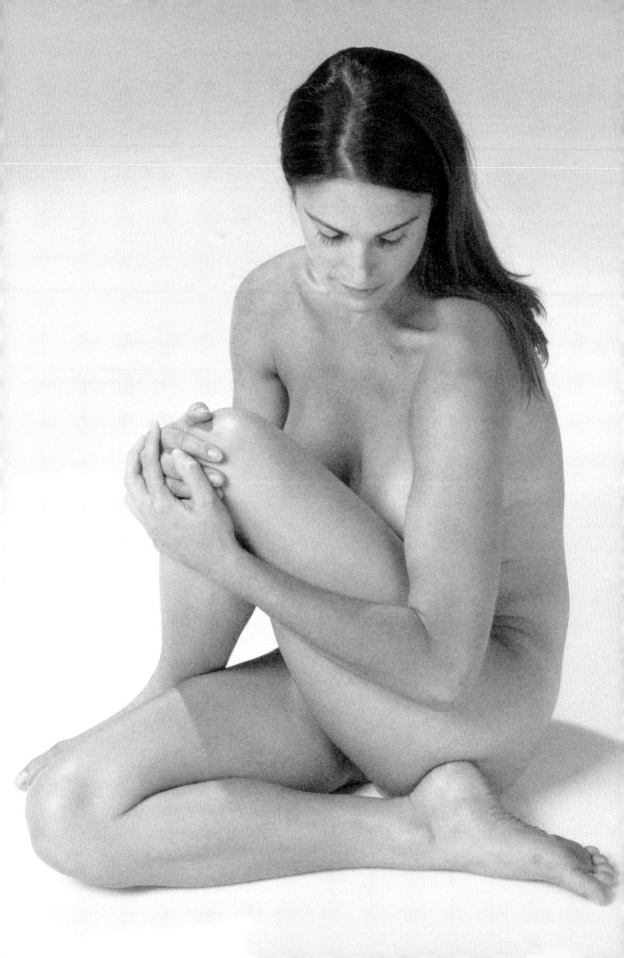

Child's Pose

Mudhasana

This is a gentle forward bend.

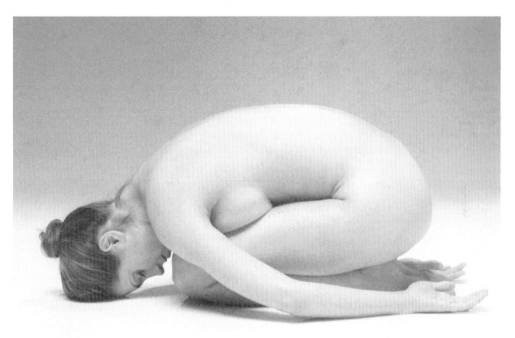

Kneel with your legs and feet together. Carefully sit back onto your heels. Slowly bend your hips forward and stretch your torso over your knees. Lengthen your spine as you rest your forehead on the floor.

You may stretch your arms overhead or let them rest by your sides as you prefer. Breathe softly and relax for ten breathes.

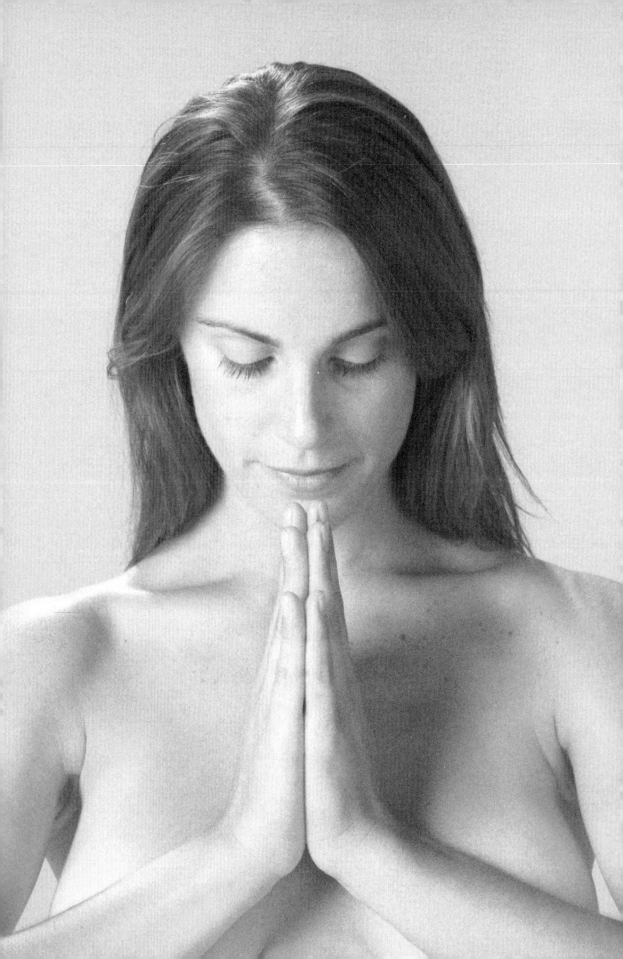

Lying-Down Spinal Twist

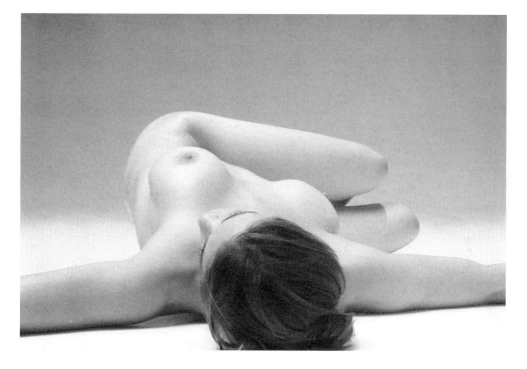

Lie flat on your back with your legs straight and feet together. Extend both arms ninety degrees out from your chest with the back of your hands resting on the floor.

Bring your knees up until the soles of your feet are flat on the floor. Keeping your legs together slowly drop your knees to the right. Turn your head to look toward your left hand. Breathe and relax for five breaths.

Raise your knees until the soles of your feet are flat on the floor and roll your head back to center. Slowly drop your knees to the left as you look toward your right hand. Ujjayi breathe and relax for five breaths.

Return to lying flat on your back. Now stretch both hands over your head as you straighten your legs back to flat on the floor.

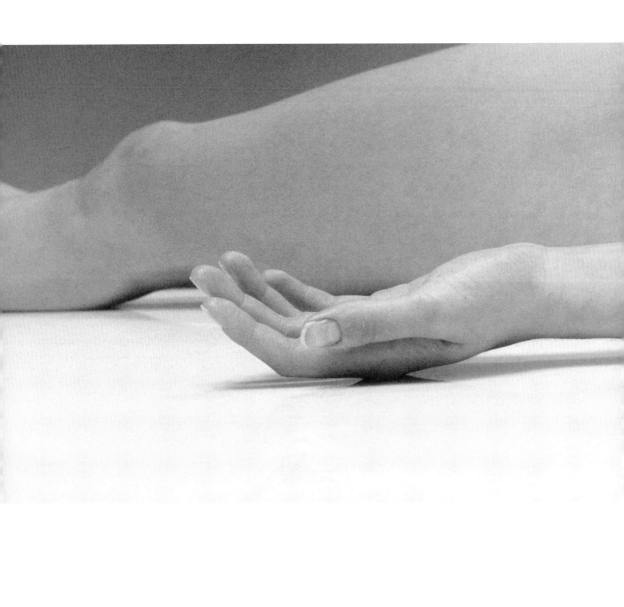

Corpse Pose

Shavasana

Lie flat on your back with your legs straight and feet apart. Let the back of your hands rest on the floor by your sides. Roll your head from side to side a few times so that it finds an easy resting place.

Relax your body beginning with feet, then ankles, legs, hips, pelvis, belly, shoulders, jaws, eyes, and scalp. Breathe softly and relax for ten to thirty minutes.

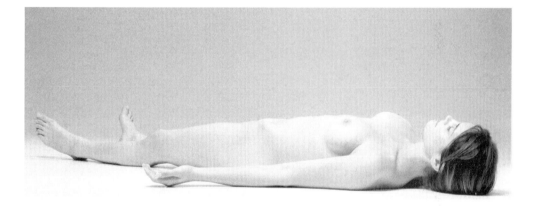

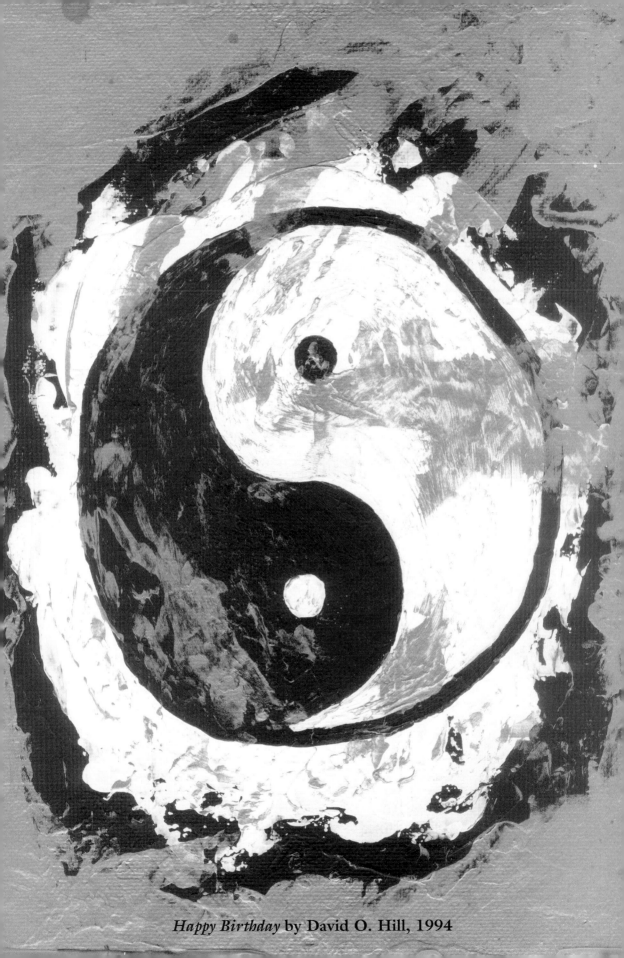

Happy Birthday by David O. Hill, 1994

CHAPTER 15

Grace

You are in a state of Grace. There exists now a perfect moment of balanced aesthetic form. This all-pervasive elegance brings pleasure to the heart, clarity of the mind, and tranquility of the soul.
—*The Illustrated I Ching*, verse 22 (Wing, translation)

Petaluma, California, Late Summer 1994: "Let's have some existential the-ater," Robert Hall suggested. We had reconvened after Sunday lunch, and I was full of stuffed grape leaves, hummus, and baba ghanouj. Drowsy with the summer heat, I waited for my coffee to kick in. Existential theater was a simple enough exercise. The group sat in a circle while someone stepped into the center. This person, without words, spontaneously acted out a personal drama with sound (no words) and movement. Stripped of words, alone, the actor tapped a raw truth underneath the often-told stories of his or her life.

The audience was simply a witness; they sat passively as the actor in the center showed a deeper self. After the theater the audience may share what they saw, cau-tioned to keep what they said objective, such as, "I saw movement that felt angry," rather than statements like, "You were angry and defiant." This taught the audience to separate what the actor does from what they, the audience, perceived about it.

Janet raised her hand, I assumed to volunteer for the exercise. She had recently become pregnant with what we already called our "Lomi baby," and had some issues with the baby's father. "Before we move into the process," Janet interjected, "I'd like to ask Alan what's on his mind. He seems distracted this weekend." I was stunned! There was something percolating at the back of my mind, but I wasn't thinking much about it. I certainly didn't think it was pressing enough to bring to the group, or for it to register with Janet.

All eyes turned to me. I was sitting next to Robert and met his gaze for a moment. He had a way of looking at me that penetrated straight to my heart. I was rarely put on the spot like this. I took a deep breath and struggled to organize my thoughts.

"I had unsafe sex with someone who is HIV positive," I blurted out. "I know it's foolish. I teach HIV-safety classes for massage therapists. I know the facts and the risks. I just got carried away in the sex. It's the stupidest thing I've done in a long time." A silence settled on the circle as the gravity of my confession registered in their minds and hearts. My eyes dropped to my hands crossed in my lap, and I felt Robert looking at me. "I've had one HIV test already. I'm still negative. I'll have another test in two months and another in six months. Most people who become HIV positive do so ninety days after exposure," I quoted from my own teacher's handout.

After too long a pause Robert said, "You've played a dangerous game of Russian roulette. You should be in the center of the circle." I took a minute to rise to my feet, stunned by the rapid-fire turn of events. My fun-loving, easygoing persona had failed me. Janet saw something more serious than even I acknowledged. I'm a natural performer who rehearsed, in my mind, imagined speeches, and possible movements to soothe away my fears: anxieties about being seen, of speaking my truth. Now I was the center of attention without a rehearsal, which was a rare and spontaneous act for me. I walked into the center of my audience.

Shoulders hunched, I stood looking at my feet. I extended my arms over my head, clasping my hands into one fist. With a bellow I dropped to my knees, slamming my fist into the mat. I roared as I pounded the mat, over and over. I vented my despair of risking my life for a cheap fuck. I finally stopped, my fists resting between my splayed knees, my lungs heaving for air. What to do now, I wondered, after this outburst and display of emotion? Wobbly, I rose and began a loose improvisation of the Five Elements of Tai chi. I extended my arms out to opposite sides, palms up, as my feet deftly glided me through a graceful circle. My ragged breath contrasted with the seamless movement. Slowly my body relaxed into the well-known forms. The rawness in my heart created new, original movements, which both soothed and thrilled me.

I peeked out at the silent eyes watching me, occasionally connecting with a safe pair of eyes. I closed the movement by turning to face Robert, kneeling and sitting back on my heels, my hands resting palm up on my thighs. Taking a deep breath I looked into Robert's eyes, stood, and returned to my seat in the circle. The audience responded with their comments, "I saw someone who was angry"; "I saw someone who was fierce, powerful, and exquisitely graceful, especially for such a large man." I listened with relaxed concentration. The uncertainty of "being on the spot" vanished, leaving me with an unusual peace of mind. Robert closed with, "I saw a man who seemed terribly shy."

> *The ancient Masters were …*
> *careful as someone crossing an iced-over stream.*
> *Alert as a warrior in enemy territory.*
> *Courteous as a guest.*
> *Fluid as melting ice.*
> *Shapeable as a block of wood.*
> *Receptive as a valley.*
> *Clear as a glass of water.*
> —*Tao Te Ching*, verse 15 (Mitchell, translation)

Grace is the third pillar, after strength and flexibility, of our body's physical foundation. Grace is often simply called balance, conscious movement, or skillful movement. *Webster's Collegiate Dictionary* defines grace as "a virtue coming from God: ease and suppleness of movement and bearing." Sitting, standing, and turning are basic movements that require grace, although we often ignore that fact and bemoan our lack of grace instead. Key to the ease and suppleness of our movements are healthy joints. There are a number of techniques that promote grace. Ballet and dance, gymnastics, yoga, or the ancient Chinese martial art of Tai chi all cultivate our body's natural ease, efficiency, and skill in moving through space.

Tai chi, like yoga, is an entire system of exercise and philosophy that works through the body, harmonizing the body, emotions, mind, and energy. In this way it is a tonic; it nurtures the whole. More than a thousand years ago, Taoist (pronounced Dow-ist) monks needed to protect themselves from violent Chinese warlords and roving bandits. The monks blended 4,000 accumulated years of Chinese healing and martial and meditative arts to create Tai chi. The synthesis of these arts includes an extraordinary number of exercises. Some are for stretching, some focus on the breath, and others are meditative.

In Tai chi the body is equally as important as the emotions, the mind and the spirit. This equality creates the harmony necessary for good health and spiritual excellence. The body becomes the fundamental foundation for the higher senses of an open heart and clear mind. Tai chi exercises, at the physical level, relax tense muscles and improve joint movement, increasing their range of motion. In traditional Chinese medicine, the health of the joints determines the amount of chi, or subtle energy, that flows through the body. The joints are the "gates" of the chi. Tight, stiff joints produce sluggish chi and dimmed vitality.

Essential to good Tai chi practice is a basic understanding of the *tan t'ien*, or *dan-tien*: the energy and gravitational center of the body located just beneath the navel. Ron Perfetti, a Tai chi teacher who lives in Hawaii, describes the importance of the *tan t'ien* in getting out of our head and into our bodies:

> *The sinking of mind is related to the idea of attention in the lower Tan T'ien, or pelvic area. This denotes the relaxing of the attention usually held in the head, shoulders, and chest, allowing it to settle down to the Tan T'ien. The result of this is a shift out of being top-heavy (and thought-oriented) into the experience of being centered (feeling/sensory-oriented).*

This shift from being "top-heavy" to "being centered" is valuable for many reasons. With all movements flowing from this powerful center of gravity, the natural alignment of the hips, pelvis, shoulders, and head are naturally aligned. It is also primary to being clear-minded. Perfetti continues:

> *The number one condition that inhibits an individual from achieving excellence in anything, including one's own health, is a state that traditional Chinese medicine refers to as being "weak-minded." This weak-minded state implies one who is easily confused, scattered, or distracted. So the first quality to be developed in Tai chi is that of strengthening one's concentration, or what is referred to in the martial arts as being centered.*

The Chinese Masters consider "being centered" the ability to focus, without distractions, on the present moment and our present experience with our complete and full attention.

Cultivating grace is important to growing consciousness for its focus on the body as it moves. Sitting meditation and the steady poses of yoga concentrate on the sensations of the body in basic stillness. Exercising grace focuses attention while we move. One of the things I love about Tai chi is that I have to pay attention. If my mind wanders I lose the flow of the Tai chi forms. I have to stop and remember where I am, regroup, and proceed. I catch my mind wandering much more quickly than in sitting meditation.

Change, as it's often said, is the one constant in the universe. Yet we humans often resist that constant change with dread. Such resistance is futile, as life has a way of crashing through our best defenses. Conscious movement helps us learn to accept change. Exercises in grace may begin as a way to increase our strength or improve our balance. But through them, change slowly becomes our friend. We find our balance in the midst of life's constant metamorphosis. And consistent exercise leads to emotional, mental, and spiritual change.

Creative strength [heaven] is within the waiting [mountain]
forming the condition for Potential Energy.
An enlightened person, therefore, is familiar with
words of the wise and the deeds of the past.
He thus nourishes his character.
—*The Illustrated I Ching,* verse 26 (Wing, translation)

Guilin, China, June 1992: "Heaven and earth," I called out. Together the group moved in silence. When our hands came to our hearts in prayer position and then separated, tracing the line of the horizon, I felt a growing sense of awe. The ancient city of Guilin lay beneath us. The massive islands of stone and trees piercing through the mists from the river below had inspired artists for thousands of years. Our rooftop perch, five stories above the city, gave us an easy view. It was truly beautiful. Adding to my awe was the juxtaposition of cultures. I was teaching a group of Chinese graduate students a simple Tai chi form. "Fire," I continued. Hands slowly met at our navels, we stepped out lifting our palms to the sun. "Water." Our palms slowly pulled the mists down over our heads.

I traveled to Hong Kong and Guilin with Ray Wright, my philosophy and world religions teacher. He was returning to China to teach a three-week class in English for graduate students at Guangxi Normal University. Four students from the University of Houston–Downtown, myself included, joined him to attend those summer classes. We were each assigned a graduate student host from the university: Wei, Benjamin, Sophie, and John Paul. They acted as translators and guides to help us with our senior project papers. My research paper involved interviewing students and townspeople to gauge "The Effects of Communism on Taoism and Buddhism in Chinese Culture." The graduate students were terrific and generous hosts.

I quickly fell into a trio with two of my fellow Americans, both named Sharon. Our dormitory was off campus near the central city. We often walked through town exploring and were quite a sight together. Sharon Attra was a short, wiry woman with a butch, blue-black, flat-top haircut. Sharon Holder-Coleman was a round, dark black woman from Jamaica with beautiful long braids. I was six-foot, four inches, 200-plus pounds, and towered over everyone. The hordes of Chinese bicyclists would slow to a crawl to gawk at the unusual sight of us walking through town.

Wei was being groomed for membership in the Communist Party. The wounds of Tiananmen Square were still fresh; our new friends were cautious of the government and careful of the sanctions imposed on all university students afterward. They could only speak honestly with us in Wei's absence. Our student hosts were each well versed in United States culture. Their grasp and depth of knowledge was incredible. They knew every bit as much about American sociology and psychology as we did (in some cases, more).

However, our Chinese hosts did not know much about Taoism or Tai chi; they considered the practices quaint and old-fashioned. I was surprised by the paradox. Our hosts could rattle on about the differences between Faulkner and Hemingway, but I met only one student who had read the *Tao Te Ching*. I was fascinated with this ancient Chinese classic text and the movements of Tai chi. A few mornings I got up very early and rode a bicycle through town to see the old men and women "dancing Tai chi" in the parks.

On a bike ride one afternoon through town, a handsome, well-dressed young man named Benjamin pulled up beside me. He asked if he could practice his English while we rode. Benjamin spoke fairly good English. After riding and talking for a while he invited me to his apartment. I was surprised to learn he lived alone in a one-room efficiency; most Chinese lived with their extended families. He worked part time as a truck driver, and most of his money went to pay his rent. I learned soon enough why his little apartment, a seeming extravagance, was a necessity.

Benjamin was gay and needed the privacy. He opened my eyes to the plight of gay people in China. Most Asian men with homosexual feelings married women to preserve the status quo of family and society. Very few identified themselves and lived openly as gay. Once arrested for indecent behavior, a gay person in China could expect years of imprisonment and hard labor. It was easier to pass as "straight" with your own wife and family. Chinese homosexuals frequented "gay hangouts" and had clandestine male love affairs on the side. Benjamin felt tormented because he knew he was gay. He didn't want a wife and family. He longed to live openly.

The day before I left Guilin, he begged to go with me. My heart ached. I knew his tears weren't for our little tryst. They were for a life of courage and freedom he dreamed of in the West. Even if he could get a visa, I knew I couldn't afford the thousands of dollars in sponsorship fees. And I couldn't afford to support him back in Houston. I was working two jobs to pay my own way through college. I did send money back to him several times to help with his junior college tuition and so he could have some fun. A hundred dollars, what I earned giving two massages, was most of a year's salary to him.

"Wood/wind,"I called out. Our little band of Chinese and American friends turned to face the river. Pushing off, we each slowly opened and made the three-quarter turn, taking in the setting sun. "Metal," I called. I focused inside myself as my scooping hands compressed into my center the beauty of China, the pleasure of my new friends, and the thrill of an adventure come true. "Tiger returns to mountain," I whispered as we wound down our exercise. We lingered on the roof, laughing, talking, and sitting on the ledge of the building as the sun sank behind the ancient mountains. Later we trailed down the steps to our final Chinese feast to wish us farewell.

I started my studies in Tai chi in the fall of 1983, when my friend J. D. and I met Tory Fritz and Kim McSherry at a book store named the Aquarian Age Bookshelf. We took beginner's classes through their Houston Institute of Astrology. Kim studied regular Tai chi classes taught by Jane Shorre in a lovely Montrose studio, and J. D. and I were soon regulars too. Afterwards we would dance our Tai chi moves across the after-hours dance floor of Rich's disco downtown (not what most Tai chi teachers have in mind for practice).

Jane was a student of Chungliang Al Huang, a dancer and Tai chi master. Chungliang is known for his love of laughter and for dancing the Tai chi forms. He seeks the inner life and spontaneity in all things.

There is a tendency in spiritual practice to focus on the minute details of a form. The forms, in turn, can become static and rigid. Chungliang tells the story of a German aristocrat who became so obsessed with his Tai chi that he lost any and all spontaneity in his movement. One day while practicing in the park, a dog walked up to the aristocrat's leg, sniffed, hiked its own leg, and peed. The man's practice was stiff as a fire hydrant.

I included the Five Elements of Tai chi in *Body Brilliance* to inspire you to with these ancient Chinese principles and exercises, as I was inspired. In describing the Five Element forms, I have been as specific about the movements as I can. There is no instruction on breathing through these forms. Let your breath happen naturally as you move, finding its own rhythm. Once you feel comfortable with the forms, let them dance through you. Play with them. Jane once called Tai chi the "Dance of the Tao." Make it so.

Tai chi Chu'an
Five Element Series

The five forms of Tai chi illustrated on the following pages are deceptively simple. The ability to perform them gracefully usually takes longer than one would think. And while the repetition of five forms might seem boring, every practice can be a new experience, like the subtle changes of the colors on the horizon. As with the other exercise routines outlined in *Body Brilliance,* to receive the greatest benefit you have to pay attention. The five forms are called:

- Tiger Returns to Mountain
- Heaven and Earth
- Fire and Water (which I have shown separately)
- Wood/Wind (demonstrated in two parts)
- Metal
- Repeat Tiger Returns to Mountain.

FURTHER READING

Huang, Chungliang Al. *Quantum Soup.* New York: E. Dutton, 1983.

Huang, Chungliang Al. *Tiger Returns to Mountain.* Moab, UT: Real People Press, 1973.

Johansen, Greg, and Ron Kurtz. *Grace Unfolding.* New York: Bell Tower, 1991.

Mitchell, Stephen. *Tao Te Ching.* New York: Harper & Row, 1988.

Perfetti, Ron. "T'ai Chi Ch'uan." Available online at www.ronperfetti.com/index. html. Downloaded Aug. 29, 2004.

Wing, R. L. *The Illustrated I Ching.* Garden City, NY: Dolphin Books, 1982.

Visit www.BodyBrillianceBook.com to download your free written copy of these exercises.

Eight forces sustain creation:
Movement and stillness,
Solidification and fluidity,
Extension and contraction,
Unification and division.

—Kabir

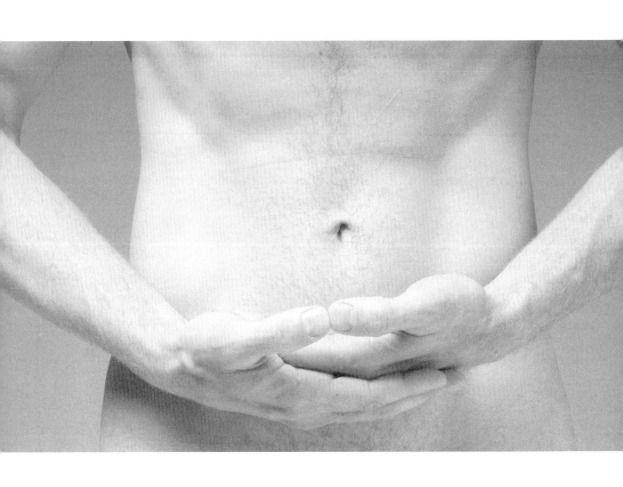

Tiger Returns to Mountain

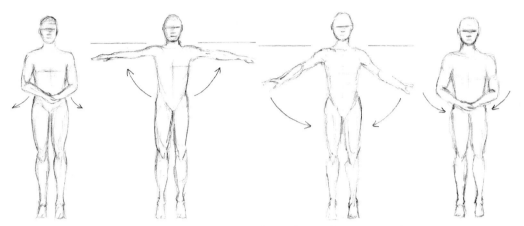

Stand relaxed with your hands cupped just beneath your navel, your center.

Slowly drop your hands down the midline of your body. At your thighs your hands flow out and up till they are shoulder height (imagine you are spreading your wings).

As your hands flow back to the midline of your body, imagine your palms scooping up the energy of the earth/mountain.

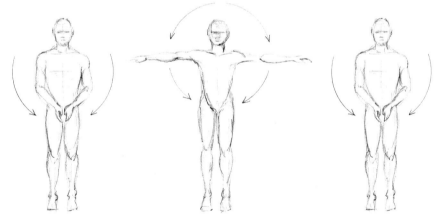

Lift your palms up through your midline. As your hands reach your face, your palms turn to face forward.

Your hands reach above your head and your arms spread out and down back to shoulder height.

Your hands continue to flow down to the midline of your body. Imagine your palms once again scooping up the energy of the earth/mountain and bringing it to your tan t'tien.

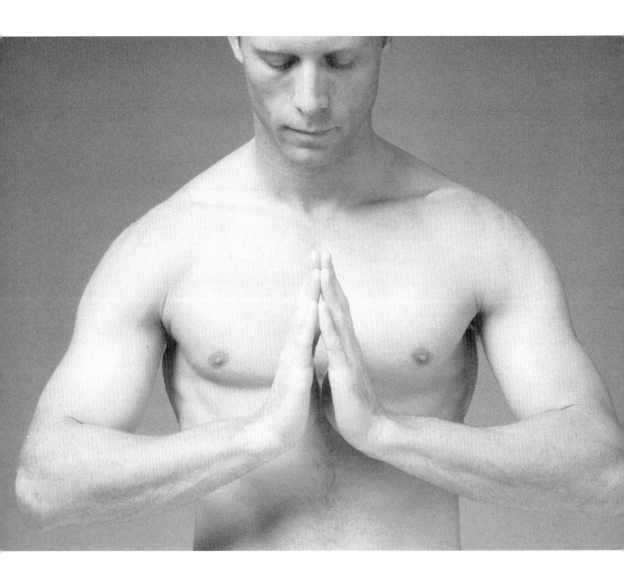

Heaven and Earth

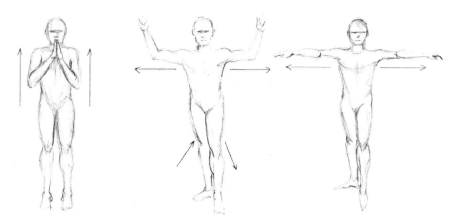

Your hands come to a soft prayer position as they reach your heart. There are two movements that happen simultaneously in Heaven and Earth. Practice each one separately, then combine them when you are ready. I have a sense of my body linked by springs and pulleys that move ever so gracefully together.

The hands move slowly from prayer position up to your throat; separating, they trace the line of the horizon.

Gently step back with your right foot. Your hips slowly shift back so that they sit directly above your right leg. Leave the ball of your left foot gently planted on the ground as you slowly lift your left heel (I like to shift my hips from side to side here to make sure I'm balanced over my right leg).

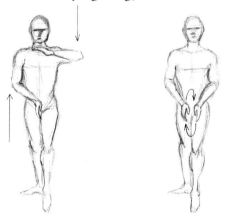

Your left hand flows above your head as your right hand flows down to your thigh; both hands rest at the midline of your body. Both hands travel your midline to meet at your center. As you approach your center, turn your palms to face each other. Imagine you are compressing the energy of heaven and earth into a ball of light.

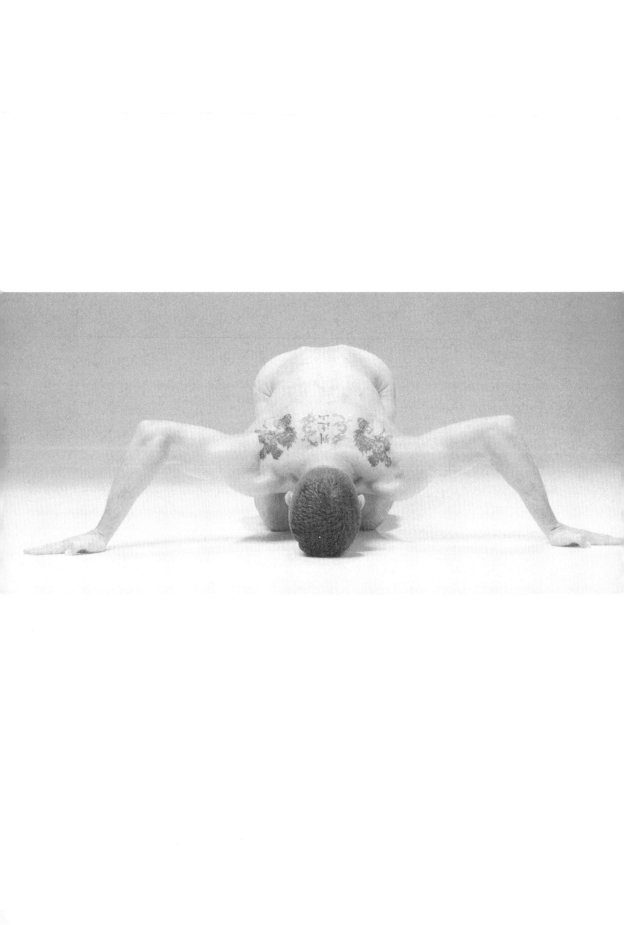

Fire

Imagine the little ball of light you were holding from Heaven and Earth. Now the fire in your belly grows to the size of a beach ball. As you reach forward, offer this large ball of light up to the sun.

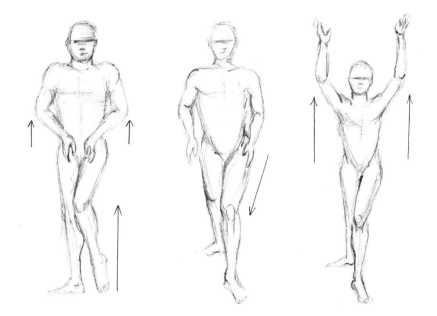

Two movements happen simultaneously. Practice each one separately. When you feel ready, combine them.

Slowly lift your left foot (which has been resting with the heel up) and take a step forward. Both feet are now planted firmly on the ground. Your hips and weight shift forward and are evenly balanced between both feet. Your torso, aligned with your center, moves forward with your hips.

Your hands pull back to your sides; your wrists rest when they brush your ribs. Pause. Gently push your arms up and away from your body until your hands, palms up, are above your head.

Tip: Be careful not to overreach. There is a tendency here to overextend the chest and reach too far forward.

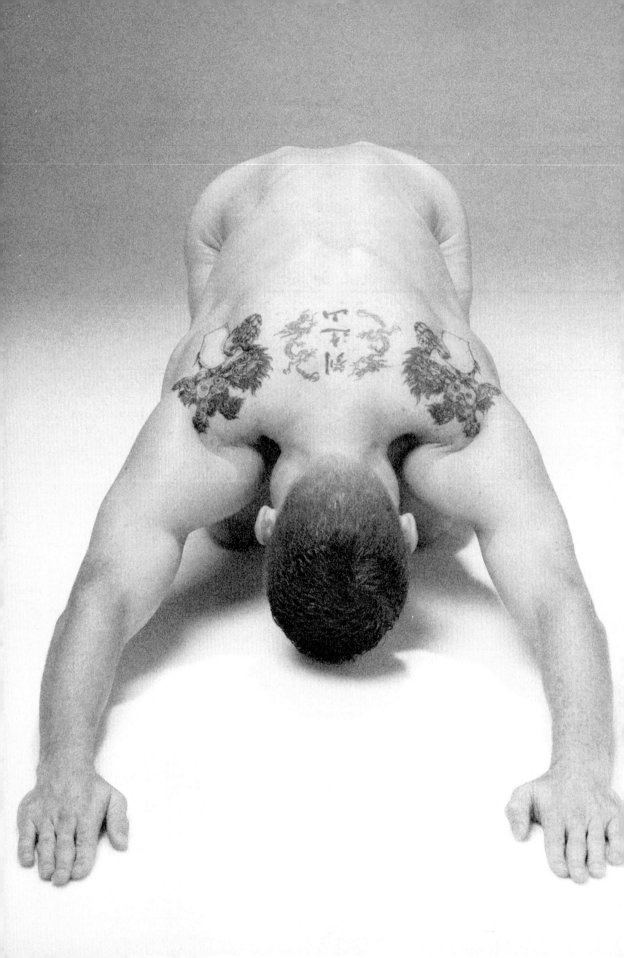

Water

Imagine, having released your fire to the sun, you are now scooping rain from the sky and drenching your body with it. As your hands caress down your body feel this water purifying and restoring you.

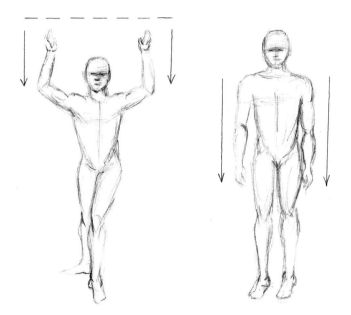

These two movements happen simultaneously in Water. Practice each one separately. When you feel ready, combine them.

Your weight shifts back and balances over your right leg. Your left foot remains gently planted on the ground.

With your elbows still up bring your forearms toward your body. Your palms automatically flip over, caressing close to your body from your head down to your thighs. Your hands rest.

I like to pause here and savor the stillness—like being washed clean after a good rain. The feeling I have during this momentary pause of the water element is emptiness: the pure potential of openness and receptivity.

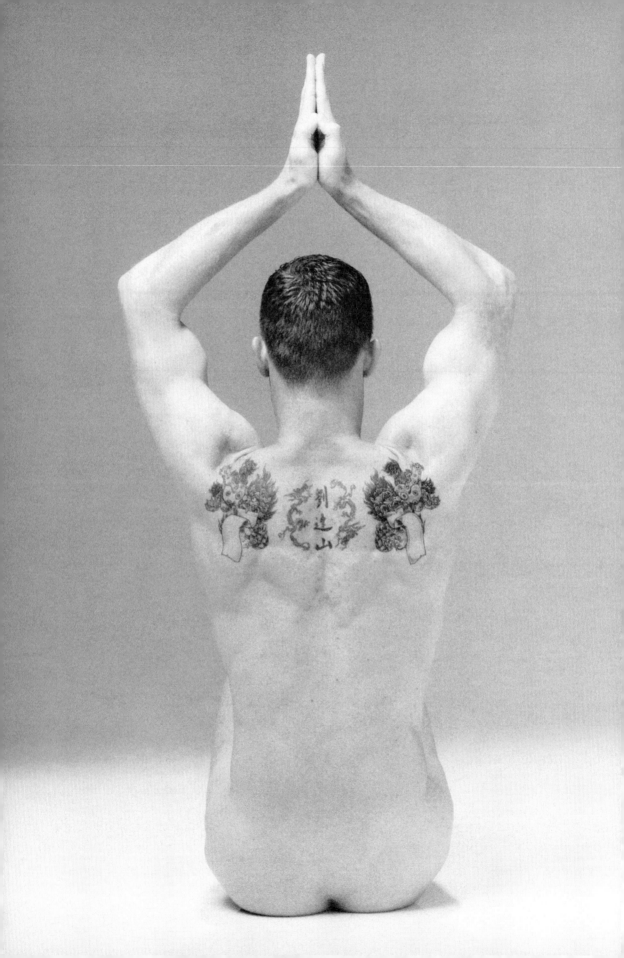

Wood/Wind Part 1

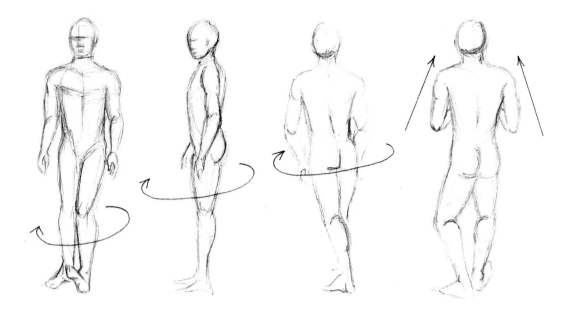

Your hands remain resting at your sides. Your weight is balanced on your right leg. Your left heel spins 90 degrees—the tips of both toes are close together. Notice the unusualness of this posture. Your right heel spins 180 degrees away from the midline of your body (clockwise). Your entire upper body follows this shift in balance. You are now fully facing the opposite wall.

Gently stretch your arms up and out from your body until your hands, palms down, are chest high.

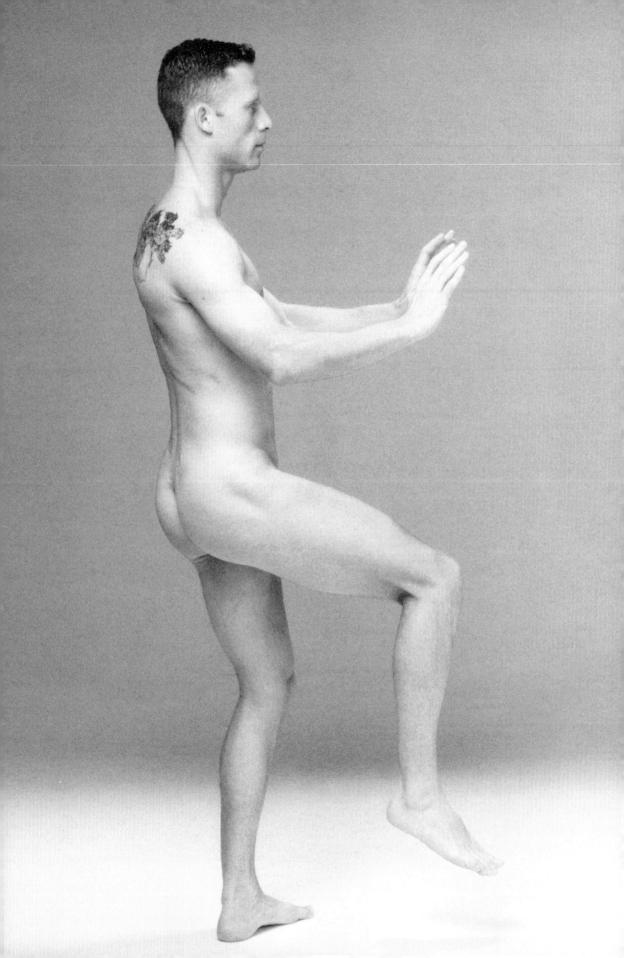

Wood/Wind, Part 2

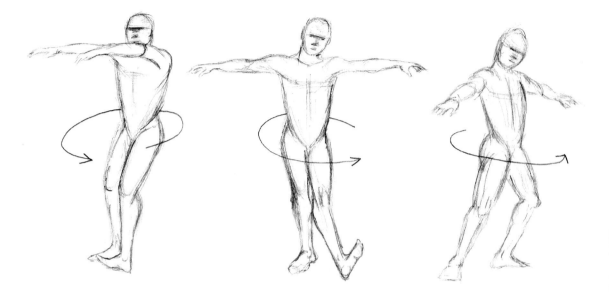

These next two movements happen simultaneously in Wood/Wind. Practice each one separately. When you feel ready, combine them.

Your right foot spins on its heel 180 degrees back toward your left foot. Notice that your toes are close together. Feel the unusualness of this posture. Your left foot turns away from your right foot 180 degrees toward front wall. Lift your right foot and turn your body counter-clockwise gently bringing your right foot so that you make a three-quarters turn.

Your arms glide apart so that they end up fully outstretched to the sides.

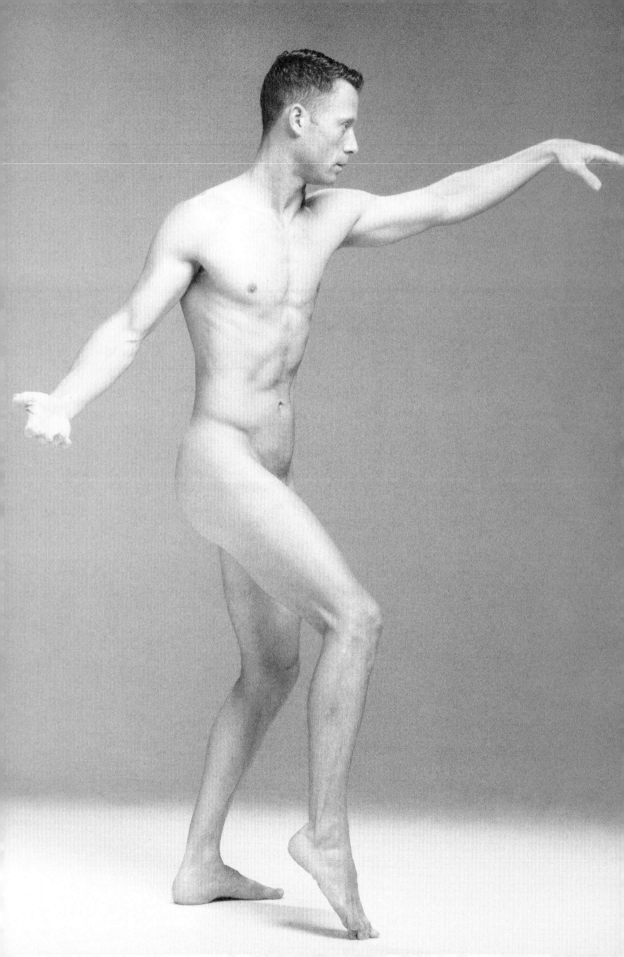

Metal

Metal is alchemy. Imagine you are scooping all the other elements of earth, fire, water, and wood/wind within your reach and compressing them into your center.

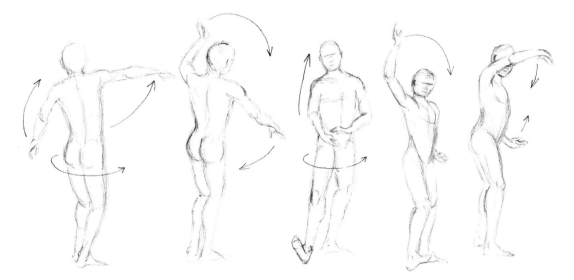

Coming off your three-quarters turn in Wood/Wind, your left foot continues an easy 60 degree spin and returns to center. Your right arm circles down so that your palm, facing up, rests under your center.

Your left hand, following the movement of your center and your left leg, reaches back and circles over your head, then drops past your face and along the midline of your body.

Your right foot spins 60 sixty degrees away from you and spins back facing the center. As your right hand circles away move your left hand, palm up, under your center.

Your right hand, following the movement of your center and your right leg, reaches back and circles over your head, then drops past your face and along the midline of your body. Imagine both of your palms compressing the energy of all these elements into the cauldron of your center. Here they meet the philosophers stone, where they are transmuted into precious metals.

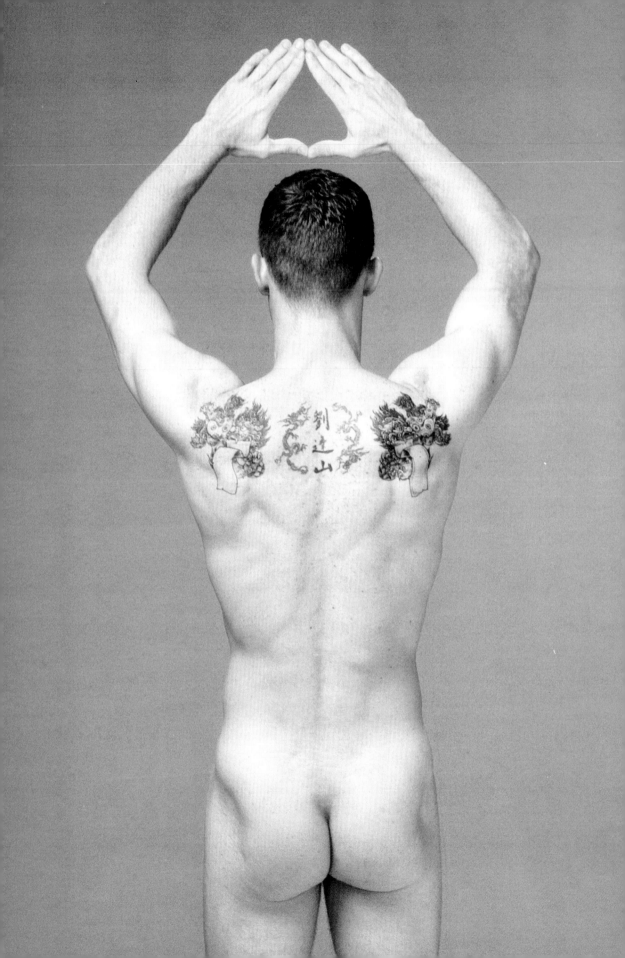

Tiger Returns to Mountain

We are right back where we started.

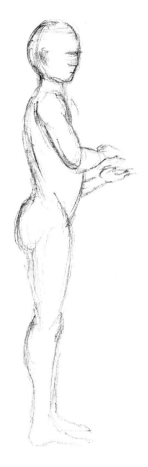

Pause for a moment to savor the alchemy of metal. Roll your top hand to rest underneath your bottom hand. Both your hands now cup the full energy of your center.

With your feet facing the wall, knees softly bent and palms cupping your center, you are in the beginning pose for Tiger Returns to Mountain.

Repeat the entire series of postures four times. You will find that you face all four directions as you do.

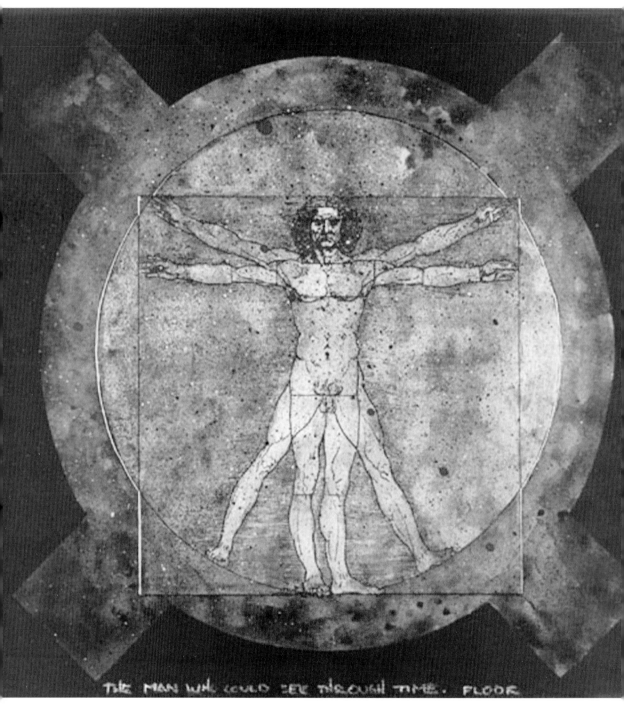

The Vitruvian Man
rendered by Keith Belli

Chapter 16

Bearing

We cannot affect one part of the body
without affecting all others.
—Joseph Heller

Petaluma, California, Late Summer 1994: Meanwhile back at the dojo, one of the students, Erika, lay shaking. Her chest, head, legs, and arms were gently vibrating, but she wasn't moving voluntarily. Her shaking came from energy moving deep inside her. Her body and her consciousness had just been touched, and the armor was dissolving.

Erika was lying on a massage table in the small sitting room of the dojo. The rest of the class huddled with just enough room for Richard to work around the table. Richard used the gentlest touch, continually calling her attention to the subtle sensations of her body: tingling, warmth, changes in her breath, the flow of emotions. As he worked he quietly told us what he was doing. "I'm moving to her chest because I can sense that there's something locked up there. I can feel that there's held energy there." He gently pressed along her rib cage to massage her diaphragm.

A classmate held her head to keep it from banging the table as her vibrations intensified. "That locked-up energy means a refusal, a no. I'm curious about the no. It's where life isn't flowing," continued Richard. "I'm encouraging life to flow there." The class was mesmerized at the scene before them. Erika's arms and legs began to thrash, and I was amazed that such a gentle touch triggered such a dramatic effect. Richard, calm and steady, directed her attention to the experience of so much energy moving. She whimpered as her legs and arms began to slow down. Over the next few minutes her jagged breathing evened, and her body stopped moving.

Suddenly peals of laughter rang out, surprising everyone but Richard. Erika's laughter trailed off into sporadic giggles. She began to talk about her mother. Richard requested her to be quiet and present in her body. Richard, talking to the class, then said, "If an emotion comes up, let the emotion out with sound or movement. Sometimes a story comes up, and we encourage the client to tell the story. Sometimes it's 'just be with the experience' and talk later. Talking can easily pull you out of the experience."

After the session Erika told us what she found so funny. "I had so many dramatic experiences with my schizophrenic mother. One day I came home to find her lying on the kitchen floor, seemingly unconscious. The garbage can was tumbled over, trash was littered about, and she had a pork-chop bone lying on top of her body. I was terrified at another episode. I caught and held my breath. Finally, my mother began to move and I realized she wasn't unconscious. Eventually I found out she was faking it to scare me. Just now on the table I laughed when I realized how absurd it all was."

Later that night a group of us went into Petaluma for Thai food. Erika looked and acted years younger; the worry lines of her face smoothed out, her eyes brightened, the laugh lines around her eyes creased with a constant smile. She was at peace.

The conversation was lively and fun, my mood high. Wayne, a great storyteller, regaled us with a tale from his years living at the San Francisco Zen Center. When the punch line came I let loose a laugh, a full satisfying belly laugh. I realized I hadn't laughed like that in way too long. It felt good.

Bearing is the stance and posture of the body in space. It is the natural alignment of the skeleton, the muscles that move the bones, and the connective tissues that stabilize them. Balance is the interplay of gravity and our bones, and a reflection of our overall sense of wholeness and ease.

My first understanding of bearing was a mishmash of memories, starting with my mother telling me, "Stand up straight. Don't slouch." I was taller than my classmates (I am six six-foot- four now), and I slumped my shoulders so as not to stand out (fat chance). And then there was my dad's military bearing from his career with the Navy. Good posture came to represent standing ramrod-straight at full attention, and that was uncomfortable for me.

Amazingly, over thousands of years of evolution, from four-legged to two-legged beings, our bones adapted to stack effortlessly one on top of the other, bringing to mind the old song "your toe bone connected to your foot bone; your foot bone connected to your ankle bone" and on up the skeletal ladder. When our bearing is good the bones are naturally aligned, the muscles are strong and relaxed, and our joints are limber. Our bodies are effortlessly balanced and our movements graceful.

When we are naturally aligned our bones create a vertical line. Our ears float over our shoulders, which float over our hips. The hips, in turn, are supported over flexible knees and strong ankles. Imagine a plumb line (or string of pearls) dropping straight down from the top of the head past our ears and through our major joints to the floor. There is a mild curve to the back of the neck and the chin is level with the ground. The lower back has a mild curve too. The chest is open with the bottom ribs pointing down to the floor, not outward.

Here's an easy self-test to check your bearing. Stand against a wall with your heels near the baseboard. If you have good posture, your sacral bone, the broad bone between your butt muscles, will touch the wall. So will your thoracic spine (the ribs behind your heart), and the back of your head, too.

The spine is especially crucial to good bearing. A healthy spine in alignment has three gentle curves that create a shallow "S." The cervical spine curves gently forward at your neck. The thoracic spine curves backward throughout the middle of your back. And then the lumbar spine curves gently forward again at your lower back. Standing against that wall, the forward curves of the neck and lower back should extend out about an inch for a person with good bearing.

Although there are myriad combinations of skeletal misalignment that can create poor posture, there are two common forms: the humpback and the swayback. A humpback slumps the mid-back, curling the shoulders and the head forward. In an attempt to counterbalance this thrust, many humpbacks will lift the chin up and out. If the chin rolls downward this posture will chronically evolve into the hunchback. If your head doesn't naturally rest against the wall in your posture self-test, it's a sign you may have humpback, or kyphosis. Notice as you bring your head to rest on the wall if your chin tilts itself up and out. This is a sign of so-called "forward head" that often accompanies humpback.

If you have more than an inch between your lower back and the wall during your self-test, then you may be swayback. Instead of the gentle curve of your lumbar spine, which should leave about an inch, you'll be able to slip the flat of your hand between your back and the wall. Swayback, or lordosis, also comes with a forward-tilting pelvis, which throws the hips off their natural vertical alignment over the knees and ankles.

Think of the differences between the Eiffel Tower and the Tower of Pisa. The Eiffel Tower sits on a solid foundation, is structurally sound, and stands tall, proud, and erect. The Tower of Pisa leans precariously, evidence of a poor foundation and a weakened structure. To save their tower from collapse, the citizens of Pisa have tried to fortify the foundation and stabilize the tilting landmark by attaching cables from the building into the ground. But the tower will never be straight.

Look at the pictures of the towers on this and on the next page and the accompanying drawings and photographs. The contrast between the soundness of the two structures is analogous to that of our own postures.

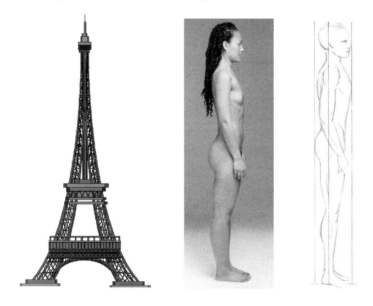

We are like the Eiffel Tower, tall and effortlessly erect, when our bones stand and move with good bearing.

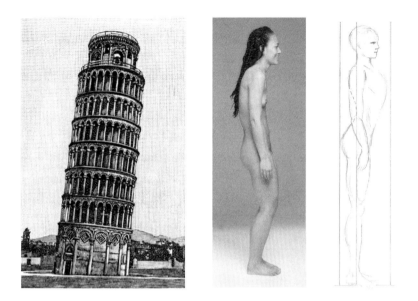

**When our posture is misaligned, we are like the Tower of Pisa,
leaning over from a weak foundation.**

When our bones stand and move with good bearing, we are like the Eiffel Tower, tall and effortlessly erect. But when our posture is misaligned, we are like the Tower of Pisa, leaning over from a weak foundation and overcompensating somewhere else in the body for that instability. Our muscles are like the cables, working overtime to realign our structure.

I sometimes joke with clients, "If the Golden Gate Bridge ever needs extra cables they can borrow the muscles in your neck."

Learning to walk will set you free.
Learning to dance gives you the greatest freedom of all:
to express your whole self, the person you are.

—Hayden

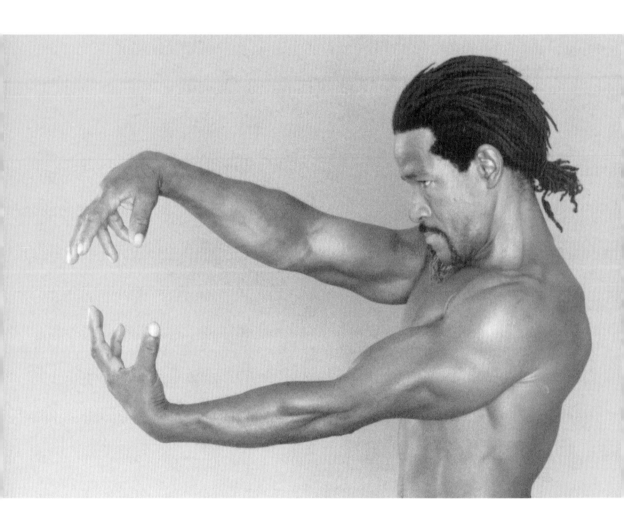

CHAPTER 17

The Connective Tissue Matrix

The living matrix is a continuous physical,
energetic, and informational network.
—James and Nora Oschman

Houston, mid-1996: Dana Sweet was working her fingers in my mouth. She pressed my gums at the base of my teeth—hard! Dana's a body-worker, and this was our seventh "Dubbing" session together. Dubbing, or Zen Bodytherapy, was a deep-tissue structural massage technique developed about 1990 by William S. "Dub" Leigh: the only person certified to practice by both Ida Rolf and Moshé Feldenkrais, another leader in the healing and human potential movement.

As she worked I tasted something unusual. At first I thought it was a mix of saliva and the latex gloves she was wearing. Strong fingers, still inside my mouth, moved to my jaw. The muscles linking my upper and lower teeth felt brittle. I had clenched my teeth and popped my jaw joints as long as I could remember. All the metham-phetamine I did during that other lifetime probably didn't help my jaws either. As Dana pressed those painful muscles, the acrid taste became stronger. It had a familiar tang but was not quite latex. In a flash I recognized it: ether! I could taste and smell the pungent gas.

A memory assembled itself in my mind. As the picture intensified the room around me slipped away. What a curious feeling, being two places at once. The present moment mingled with the distant past, when I was five years old. I was lying on a hospital gurney. My grandmother was a nurse. She was dressed for surgery and held my hand. The mask and cap hid her face; all I could see were her blue eyes framed by familiar cat-eye glasses. A green smock hid the crisp nurse's uniform I had seen her wear to work that morning. The lights shined brightly above her head.

I was not afraid. Nanny, as I knew her, told me everything would be okay, she would be with me the whole time the doctor operated on me. She said she loved me, and that when I woke up my tonsils would be gone. A mask was placed over my face and I smelled the ether. Nanny told me to take deep breaths. I looked into her eyes and saw the comfort and love she had for me (it was the same comfort and love that sustained me through many a difficult day). I trusted her and knew that "everything will be okay." I counted backward: 100, 99, 98, 97, and at 92, I gently nodded off to sleep.

Back in Houston, with Dana's fingers in my mouth, I coughed and spit with the taste of ether.

How did Richard's gentle touch cause Erika's body to shake so dramatically? How do emotions become "armored" into our muscles, to use Wilhelm Reich's idea? How did the muscles of my mouth store the memory of a long-ago tonsillectomy? The answer is connective tissue. All the cells and tissues of our body are interconnected, networked together by a "connective tissue matrix," or CT matrix.

Most people know about tendons and ligaments, the more common connective tissues; however, connective tissues stretch from within each cell and throughout every single organ of the body. Microscopic fibers of connective tissue, known as the cytoskeleton, shape each cell. Those fibers interlace with the cell wall, which is also partially made up by connective tissue. Groups of cells are bound together with connective tissue.

Within the muscles, microscopic strands of connective tissue intertwine with the muscle fibers. These strands are bundled together by larger sheets of connective tissue to form entire muscles. Then the muscular system is covered in fascia, the large envelope of connective tissue that allows the muscles to glide over each other (it's also that ribbon of fat in a beefsteak that makes meat tender). The muscles are attached to bones by connective tissues called tendons. Ligaments stabilize joints and bones. Connective tissue lines all the body's cavities and surrounds every internal organ.

Every cell and organ in the entire body is part of a complex network of connective tissue fibers. According to an article in *Massage Therapy Journal* by James and

Nora Oschman, "the organs, tissues, cells, organelles, including the nucleus, and the strands of genetic material, DNA, can be viewed as a continuous and unbroken fabric: a matrix within a matrix within a matrix." The CT matrix, along with our bones, gives our bodies their shape and structure.

So how does the CT matrix store memories? It is one of the body's three primary communication systems; the other two are the endocrine system and the nervous system. The CT matrix is ultra-sensitive to pressure, sensation, and intense emotions, and these stimuli are sensed as vibrations that are conducted throughout the matrix. The endocrine system relies on hormones to send messages to the body, while the nervous system uses electrical impulses much like a telegraph.

When one area of the body feels sensation, that vibration ripples through the whole matrix. The CT matrix not only conducts the vibrations of our physical experience but also records them. Intense experiences, both joyous and traumatic vibrations, are stored in the CT matrix. The most intense memories are stored in the deeper muscle groups of the body. That's how deep-tissue touch can release long-forgotten memories and feelings.

The CT matrix plays a major role in the peaking of vital physical intelligence for a number of reasons. Your posture is one measure of the health of your connective tissues, which are, by nature, flexible. Stress of any kind tightens the connective tissues, and chronic contractions in the CT matrix tighten the muscles and joints. If the tensions are held for too long they gradually stiffen and distort the body's natural posture. Long-held chronic stress and injury establish new patterns of posture and movement. Eventually, skewed posture limits the body's full range of motion, making the body and its systems inefficient.

Thomas Hanna, a somatic movement therapist, spotlighted several types of poor posture. He based these postures on some of the body's natural reflexes, no different than your knee jerking when the doctor taps it with a rubber hammer. Hanna recognized that all the body's reflexes are necessary for total function.

However, some people do not relax after the need for that reflex has passed. They unconsciously hold on to the tightened muscles for the extra sense of safety they feel. The tightening of the reflex becomes a habit that slowly but surely distorts the body's posture. That slow degeneration of good posture leads to other chronic pains and ailments.

Hanna identified the "red-light posture," or our retreat response, as one of the body's reflex reactions to stress. When humans feel anxious, whether vaguely apprehensive or frightened of real danger, they tighten their gut muscles, as if the muscles are expecting a blow of some kind. "When you touch a sea anemone, its circle of small tentacles quickly retracts, withdrawing from the threatening stimulus," said Hanna, drawing a parallel.

However, chronically tightening the gut—being ever on guard—tilts the pelvis and pulls the shoulders back, which in turn skews the entire alignment of the other bones. Additionally, tight abs compress the abdominal organs and shorten breath. The chronic red-light reflex eventually leads to a swayback posture and is responsible for many of the ailments associated with old age. With the gut tightened the chest puffs out, giving an impression of false bravado. Habitually raised shoulders (what I call "Joan Crawford padded shoulders") are also a symptom of the red-light reflex. The puffed-out chest and raised shoulders tilt the neck and chin up and out. After years of carrying the body in such a skewed posture, the muscles scream out in pain.

The "green-light posture" reflex is another of the body's responses to stress. If the red-light response is to retreat, the green-light response is to act. Hanna noted that this reflex starts at the age of five to six months when a baby arches its back, straightens its knees, and lifts its head forward (the Landau reflex). Self-propulsion is the natural effect of the green-light reflex and is necessary to our ability to stand and move. For those people who cannot relax after this reflex, who habitually put the call to movement and action on hold, their bodies harden into a slump-back posture: a stoop with the back lifted and arched. This posture is the prime culprit of the bad-back epidemic.

Gravity—it's not just a good idea. It's the law.

—Virginia Platts

The following photographs contrast natural, erect posture against the most common forms of poor posture—and show us how good posture went bad.

The Red-Light Reflex and Swayback: Notice the hips are pressed back and the chest thrust out. This posture reflects a personality always "on guard."

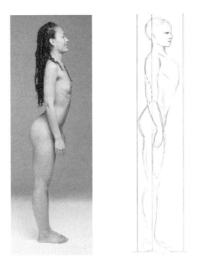

The Green-Light Reflex and Humpback: Notice the hips are tilted back and the lower back pressed forward as the shoulders stoop and the chin points up and out. This personality type tends to have poor personal boundaries and perhaps low self-esteem.

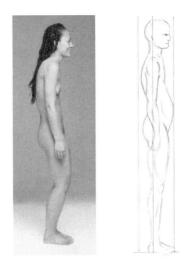

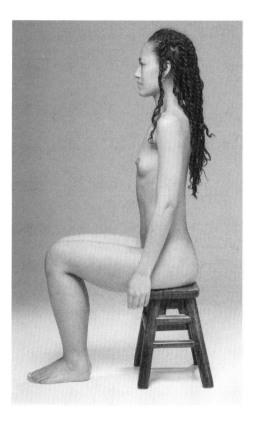 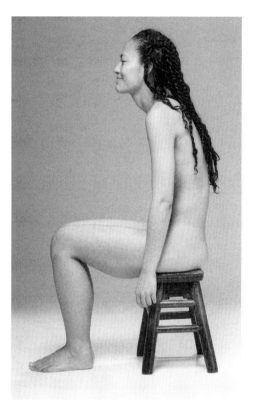

The body aligned while sitting.   The body poorly aligned while sitting.

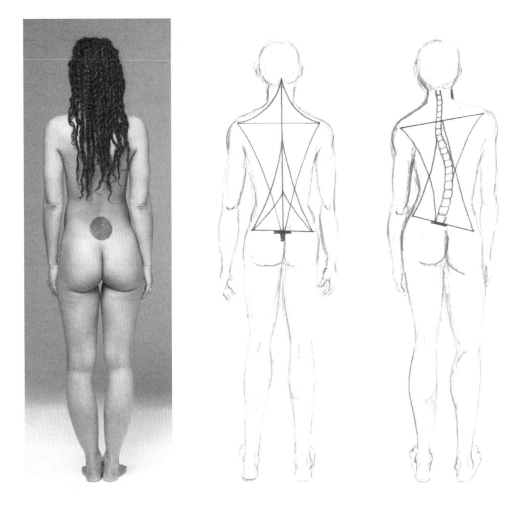

The body standing
in alignment.

The spine misaligned.

FURTHER READING

Oschman, James and Nora. "Somatic Recall," parts 1 and 2. *Massage Therapy Journal*, Summer and Autumn 1995.

*Do not lose your knowledge that man's proper estate
is an upright posture, an intransigent mind,
and a step that travels unlimited roads.*

—Ayn Rand

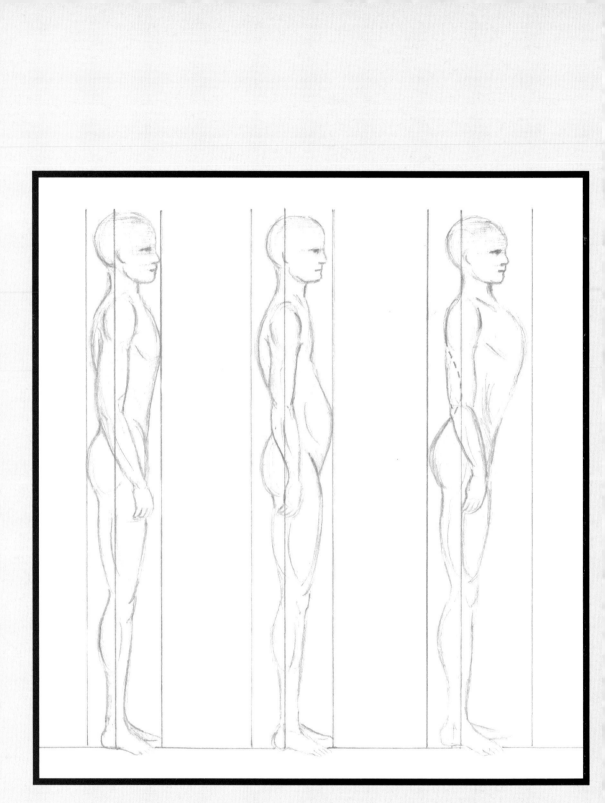

The Body Aligned   The Body Humpbacked   The Body Swaybacked

CHAPTER 18

Structural Integration

*[Rolf] created a technique that uses the reorganization of
human anatomy not only to better health but also
to reach higher states of consciousness.*
—Karen Lackritz

Many postural or skeletal imbalances can be corrected by deep-touch massage. Once the connective tissue contracts it can be softened and stretched out again. It may take some time, however, depending on the rigidity of the tension held and the length of time the tissue has been inflexible.

Massage is well known for its therapeutic and relaxing benefits. Superficial massage techniques like Swedish have a gentle relaxing effect on the body but have little effect on posture. The deep-tissue structural modalities like Rolfing, LomiWork, Hellerwork, and Zen Bodytherapy (Dubbing) are designed to affect our posture, the CT matrix and our life's vitality. Deep-tissue work is called "structural alignment" because it affects the posture of the skeletal system; the fascia, tendons, and ligaments, and the adhesions, or "knots," in the muscle tissues. Creating change in one area generates subtle effects throughout the whole system.

Structural Integration, or Rolfing, is the most famous of the deep-tissue alignment schools. As I outlined in Chapter Eight, Rolfing is a series of ten bodywork sessions, each of which focuses on different parts of the body. Following a photographic assessment of the client's posture and other imbalances, the therapist starts by working on the chest to relax the client's breathing, then moves to the feet, ankles and legs to establish a stable foundation. Work on the pelvis creates a base for the torso and arms. Moving up through the shoulders and neck the head is straightened, and final photographs reveal the improved posture.

The relation between the body and the unconscious mind is often dramatically revealed during these sessions. Memories and emotions can flood the mind, and important shifts in thinking and behavior can occur as a result of this therapy. Robert Hall, of the Lomi School, teaches that the microscopic level of connective tissue is the interface between our thinking mind and our physical bodies.

Repetitive thinking shows up in the tissues of our bodies as repetitive habits of moving and holding. If our thought patterns are fearful and painful, the connective tissues will contract, which distorts the carriage of the bones. If the thought patterns are open and expansive, the connective tissue remains flexible and the body balanced and poised. Caroline Myss, Ph.D., the medical intuitive and bestselling author, puts it this way, "Your biography [what you think and how you feel about your life] becomes your biology."

I finally signed up for a Rolfing series with Deborah Starrett, a certified Rolfer. At my first session she took a number of Polaroid photos of me in my underwear. Using the photographs she pointed out how my body was swayed, twisted, and bowed. I had fooled myself in the mirror, thinking I had pretty good posture. She acknowledged that, "These are not things most people would notice walking down the street." Under Deborah's scrutiny I realized how distorted my body was. During the Rolfing series I could feel my body changing, as well as see it changing, thanks to more Polaroids.

However, the most dramatic change I noticed was in my attitude. By now my business, Essential Touch, was a well-established massage therapy clinic. My private practice was quite successful, and I subleased massage rooms to other therapists. But I was burned out. When I rented a room to a therapist I made clear that my role as a landlord was to provide a clean professional clinic and offer some guidance. Essential Touch would, from time to time, refer overflow clients to them, but they were responsible for growing their own massage practice. Unfortunately, some of the therapists expected me to provide more than the occasional client.

As my Rolfing sessions progressed, I stood taller. My legs and feet walked directly forward instead of splaying outward. I grew more confident as my body moved with ease. I felt better. At the office I decided to cut through all the misplaced expectations, telling myself over and over, "My life could be easy; no more hassles." A few months after the Rolfing series ended I completely reassessed my priorities. I rented a one-man studio in the Montrose area for my private practice and closed the clinic.

The first thing I consider when choosing a deep-tissue bodyworker is his or her ability to be "present": what I call the "gift of presence." Presence of mind signals clarity of the spirit in the practitioner. It demonstrates the growth of consciousness in his or her life. Robert Hall described presence as being awake. With the "gift of presence," a safe place for emotional work is easily created. The therapist has an increased ability to accept any and all of the emotions and experiences that might arise during a session.

Presence mirrors a higher vibration of inner vitality. Do you remember the capacity of the connective tissue matrix to conduct vibrations throughout the entire body (Chapter Seventeen)? If your therapist works with presence, then the frequency vibration of his or her touch is greater. You experience more. Richard Strozzi HecklerStrozzi-Heckler writes:

> *What we actually have to offer another is the simple but daring contribution of our genuine presence. Techniques and theories abound and we can learn half a dozen in an hour, but it is in the pulsing contact between living things that healing and beauty take place. Presence is being present—a state pregnated with an open-ended curiosity, relaxation, and power that comes from seamlessly knitting together one's mind, body and spirit.*

The schools of deep touch have a reputation for being painful, and some of the sessions are indeed intense. A gifted therapist will work to the edge of your discomfort and then pause. With attention and conscious breathing the muscles and fascia often "melt" to allow a deeper touch. Real emotional and psychic transformations skate on the edge of pain and discomfort. If a therapist attempts to slam through the painfully tight muscles to the inner core, the body contracts along with the psychic and emotional energies. If the body is contracting in pain, there is no way for the tension, energy, or emotions already held in the muscles to be released. It is in respecting the pain thresholds that trust and respect are gained. The emotions are freed and expressed, and the muscles can permanently release their tension.

Many Westerners have poor boundaries. We learn early in life to endure more pain than we should tolerate. In general, we don't know how to say, "This hurts; this is enough for this time, in this place." We also don't expect to have our boundaries respected. Honoring another's pain threshold can have immediate and lifelong benefits.

I always gave away too much of myself. I was one of those guys who would bankrupt myself financially, emotionally, and physically before I reached my limits, before I even realized I was in "the red." I just gave and gave, believing that if I said, "No. That's enough!" people wouldn't like me. It sounds silly now, but in those days I was really afraid of losing friends for "just saying no."

Ann Lasater, my first teacher in LomiWork, often talked of the importance of saying, "That's enough" in our sessions, of riding the edge of the pain threshold. When I received bodywork on her table I would tighten up in pain and endure the pressure until she stopped. She was quite skilled at reading my body and lightening up the pressure if I contorted in pain.

One day before a session she specifically asked me to watch my pain threshold and to tell her the second I felt my body contracting in pain. I agreed. While she was working on my shins, I felt the pain. I held off saying anything for a few minutes, and then blurted out shrilly, "That's enough." Ann eased her touch as she continued to work my leg. I relaxed deeply, both my leg and my mind. Later in the session Ann worked my shoulder. When the pain hit, I said more quietly, "That's enough." She eased the pressure and continued to work.

By paying attention, Ann established a simple respect for the limits of my body: no coercion, no manipulation, and no agenda. I never remembered saying "No" before and being heard and respected. With Ann there was no backlash. Now I knew there was at least one person in this world who would respect me and my "No." This was a life-turning lesson for me. From that revelation on the massage table, I sheepishly began to say "No" in other areas of my life. It became a game and a lifelong exercise for me. Now I enjoy saying, "No, thank you."

There are thoughts which are prayers.
There are moments when, whatever the posture of the body,
the soul is on its knees..

—Victor Hugo

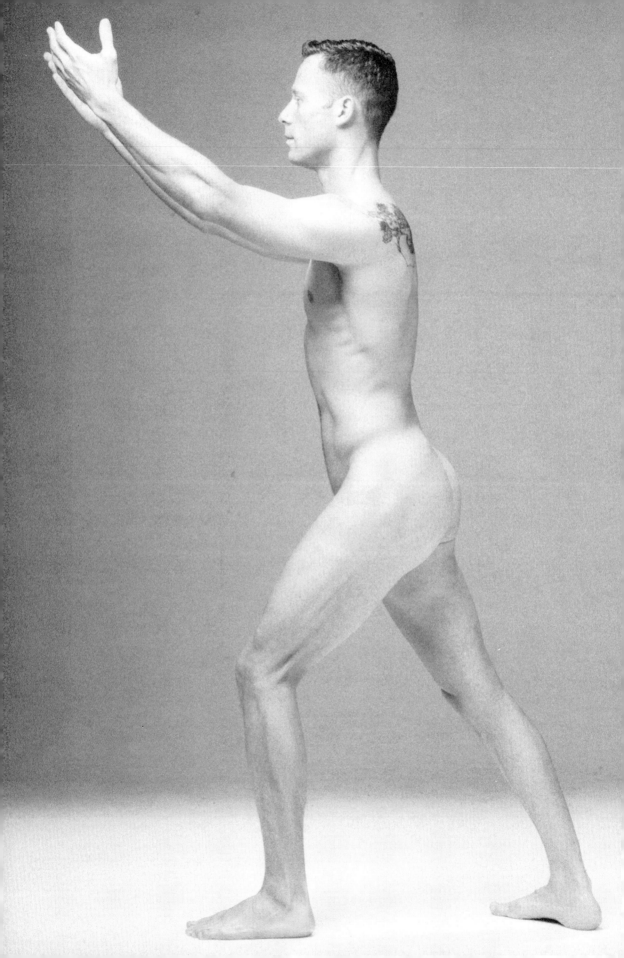

CHAPTER 19

The Body Brilliant Sessions

If you believe you can or if you believe
you can't ... you're right!
—Henry Ford

The Body Brilliant Sessions, like many innovations, are the result of a "blinding flash of the obvious." They integrate my years of diverse training to combine Applied Kinesiology, PSYCH-K, Polarity Therapy and Somatic deep-tissue massage (simplified Rolfing) into a thorough body/heart/mind/spirit treatment.

Each Body Brilliant session focuses on one of the five elements of polarity therapy: earth, water, fire, air, and ether. Each session also focuses on one of the seven bands of armored muscle tissues identified by Wilhelm Reich: eyes, jaws, neck, chest, diaphragm, belly, and pelvis (and I've added feet and legs). The intent is to release negative belief patterns, free the movement of energy through the body's energy grid, and melt the armored muscle and connective tissues. The sessions last about two hours, as we cover a lot of territory in that time. I have divided the work into ten sessions. They are not a series but individual, directed therapies. The sessions and their components are listed below, followed by an examination of the different disciplines in more detail.

Applied Kinesiology

Kinesiology, or the study of movement in relation to human anatomy, has its roots in the early 1960s with Dr. George Goodheart, D.C. an American chiropractor. Goodheart correlated the relationship among internal organs, acupuncture meridians, and skeletal muscles. He realized that the skeletal muscles, like the acupuncture meridians, are a way to monitor the functions of our internal organs. He called this work applied kinesiology.

Then, in the early 1970s, another chiropractor, John Thie, systematized kinesiology for the lay person, making the techniques simple and practical for anyone to learn. He wrote the book *Touch for Health* and began teaching. Since then Thie's system has been taught in over fifty countries and his book translated into many languages.

Of the many advances in applied kinesiology, the most well-known is muscle testing, a test that measures the feedback loop between the nervous system and the skeletal muscles. A typical muscle testing procedure goes as follows: an examiner will likely use the straight-arm test on a deltoid muscle to evaluate how well the muscle resists an external push. If the muscle is capable of "resisting," then the examiner can proceed with a second muscle test to check the status of almost any neurological or physiological event in the body: physical, chemical, emotional, a belief, or a memory.

Muscle testing also measures the feedback loop between the nervous system, the skeletal muscles, and the subconscious mind. When used properly muscle testing can be an accurate detector of subconscious truths. Because the subconscious mind controls motor functions in the body such as muscle movement, we can use this "built in" biofeedback test to find out whether the subconscious agrees or disagrees with a given belief statement.

PSYCH-K

Your life is a reflection of your beliefs. These beliefs (usually subconscious) represent the cumulative effect of lifelong "programming." As a result of our past negative programming, we sometimes think and behave in self-defeating ways. PSYCH-K helps us communicate directly with both the super-conscious and the subconscious minds and provides a user-friendly way to change negative beliefs into positive, supportive ones.

Changing subconscious beliefs that sabotage well-intentioned actions is similar to reprogramming a personal computer. Using PSYCH-K balances—a kind of "mental keyboard"—you can, in effect, write new software for your own brain. With PSYCH-K you can increase cross talk between the two brain hemispheres, thereby achieving a more whole-brained state—ideal for changing subconscious beliefs. In addition, when the right and left hemispheres of the brain are in simultaneous communication, the qualities and characteristics of both hemispheres are available to maximize your full potential to face life's challenges.

Only your beliefs set the limits of what you can achieve. Employing PSYCH-K techniques to deal with the powerful subconscious mind, "We have the capacity to consciously evaluate our responses to environmental stimuli and change old responses any time we desire … We are not stuck with our genes or our self-defeating behavior!" exults Bruce Lipton, Ph.D., in his book *Biology of Belief.*

PSYCH-K is a blend of various tools for change, some contemporary and some ancient. This unique process, originated by Rob M. Williams, was the result of years of research and thousands of sessions with individuals and groups. Changing our subconscious beliefs and directing our lives to our dreams gives truth to Otto Rank's quote, "What we achieve inwardly will change outer reality." It also emphasizes the important and powerful combination of positive beliefs plus conscious awareness.

Polarity Therapy

The human energy field is described in many sources, both ancient and modern. According to polarity therapy, our physical, psychological, and spiritual well-being depends on the free and uninterrupted flow of this "life energy" around and through the body. The term "polarity" refers to the universal pulsation of expansion/contraction or repulsion/attraction known as yin and yang.

This life-force energy, which is comparable to chi in traditional Chinese medicine and prana in the Ayurvedic discipline, is said to move in currents between a positive and negative pole. The pulse, which always passes through a neutral position, creates the energetic "template" for the physical body. Interruption of this flow is thought to lead to pain and illness. Polarity therapists use bodywork, diet, exercise, and self-awareness to help restore and balance a person's energy flow so that the body can heal itself naturally.

As detailed in Chapter Eight, Polarity Therapy was developed by Dr. Randolph Stone, who conducted a thorough investigation of energy in the healing arts over the course of his sixty-year medical career. Drawing on information from a wide range of sources, including his lifelong studies of Eastern medicine, Stone found that the human energy field is affected by touch, diet, movement, sound, attitudes, relationships, life experience, trauma, and environmental factors. Polarity therapy lends an energy-based perspective to these subjects.

Somatic Deep-Tissue Massage

Somatic massage is more than just a type of deep-tissue massage. The therapy synthesizes the client's awareness, thereby enabling the release of long-held tension and the alignment of body/mind/spirit. Many imbalances—even disabilities—can be corrected by deep-touch massage.

Somatic massage seeks to correct and realign posture and the body's musculature by working to stretch the connective tissues. Even though the connective tissue may have contracted, it can be softened and stretched out again. Therapy could take some time, depending on the tension and rigidity of the tissues and the length of time the muscles have been inflexible.

Encouragingly, creating change in one part of the body or mind generates subtle changes throughout the whole system. Massage is well known for its therapeutic and relaxing benefits, but the relationship between the body and the unconscious mind has been dramatically revealed during these deep-tissue somatic massage sessions. Memories and emotions flood the mind. Patients experience important shifts in thinking and behavior, breaking through Wilhelm Reich's rigid "armoring" to release long-repressed disappointments and anxieties.

Some of us are lucky enough to regain a portion of the flexibility we once enjoyed. And some of us finally let go, opening our hearts to the pure pleasure of life that I saw expressed at recess on a school playground in Houston.

For any one technique or combination of therapies to accomplish such miracles is a tall order. But I've seen the results of conscious, attentive bodywork. I'm living proof.

Mirror Affirmations

Mirror affirmations are the homework assignment after each Body Brilliant session. The balances are an excellent way to free energy in the body/mind/spirit, but we still have to build the new neural pathways in the brain to make our potential a reality in the world. The affirmations help to anchor in the balances and to create the progress we most want for our lives.

The mirror affirmations and the Level One Symbols are based on the work of Dawn Clark, a twenty-first century shaman and author of *Gifts for the Soul* and *The Gifts in Action*. The affirmations are simple, positive, present, personal, and dynamic.

The integration of Dawn Clark's symbols is what makes these affirmations so effective.

Below is an example of a person's energy body prior to and immediately after drawing the Level 1 symbols.

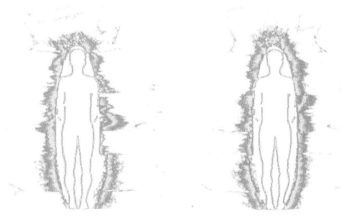

| Before Images | After Images |

Opening the energy allows the conscious mirror work to help build new neural pathways in the brain and integrate your new belief statement into subconscious, conscious, and super-conscious minds. This in turn creates your newly balanced belief into three-dimensional reality.

Visit www.dawnclark.net/symbols.htm to download your free symbols.

Step 1: On a clean white sheet of paper write down your affirmations. These affirmations are dynamic, first person, and present tense. Here's an example: I attract

my perfect lean and healthy body by weighing _____ pounds and having a _____%
body fat ratio. And I choose to let it be fast, fun, and easy.

Step 2: Underneath your affirmations, draw the three symbols from *Gifts for the Soul*, from right to left on a clean white sheet of paper.

Step 3: Affirm — Mirror Affirmations based on *The Gifts in Action*.

Stand twelve to eighteen inches from a mirror in a location with enough light to see the pupils of your eyes. Focus on the left eye, the window to the logical, linear, left side of your brain. State positive affirmations, using your own name, and repeat three times for each affirmation or until you believe what you're saying.

Write them down if it helps.

The Ten Body Brilliant Sessions

Session 1: Earth

- Step 1: PSYCH-K balance

- Step 2: Deep polarity points/Minor Foot points

- Step 3: Deep massage: Top and bottom of feet

- Step 4: Gentle polarity: Coccyx to axis/earth element/close

- Step 5: Mirror affirmations

Session 2: Extended earth

- Step 1: PSYCH-K balance

- Step 2: Deep polarity points/Minor leg points

- Step 3: Somatic deep massage: Legs/side, front and back

- Step 4: Gentle polarity: extended earth/close

- Step 5: Mirror affirmations

Session 3: Water

- Step 1: PSYCH-K balance

- Step 2: Deep polarity points

- Step 3: Dry body brushing/Lymphatic essential oils
- Step 4: Lymphatic massage
- Step 5: Water element/Pubic area to clavicle X 2/close
- Step 6: Mirror affirmations

Session 4: Extended water

- Step 1: PSYCH-K Balance
- Step 2: Deep polarity points
- Step 3: Deep massage: Belly/Soft diaphragm/Low back
- Step 4: Extended water element/Pubic to clavicle X 2/close
- Step 5: Mirror affirmations

Session 5: Fire

- Step 1: PSYCH-K balance
- Step 2: Deep polarity points
- Step 3: Belly, diaphragm, side-lying back
- Step 4: Fire element
- Step 5: Cellular reformatting
- Step 6: Mirror affirmations

Session 6: Extended fire/crown

- Step 1: PSYCH-K balance
- Step 2: Deep polarity points
- Step 3: Eyes/Face/Scalp/Crown
- Step 4: Extended fire element/Close
- Step 5: Mirror affirmations

Session 7: Air

- Step 1: PSYCH-K balance
- Step 2: Deep Polarity points/Minor arm points

- Step 3: Diaphragm/Chest/Front of arms
- Step 4: Gentle polarity: clavicle to ribs/Air element
- Step 5: Mirror affirmations

Session 8: Extended Air

Energy test: Sympathetic nervous system, para-sympathetic nervous system, or both

- Step 1: PSYCH-K balance
- Step 2: Deep polarity points
- Step 3: Full back: Back of arms/Child's pose/Cobra
- Step 4: Sympathetic or para-sympathetic nervous system
- Step 5: Mirror affirmations

Session 9: Ether

- Step 1: PSYCH-K balance
- Step 2: Deep polarity points
- Step 3: Neck/Shoulder nine points/Soundings
- Step 4: Ether element
- Step 5: Mirror affirmations

Session 10: Extended Ether: The chakras

- Step 1: PSYCH-K balance
- Step 2: Deep polarity points
- Step 3: Deep massage: neck/jaws
- Step 4: Chakra balance/Close
- Step 5: Mirror affirmations

Your innate body wisdom (also called your higher self or super-consciousness) directs the sessions through energy and muscle testing, also known as applied kinesiology. Your body wisdom guides us to determine what it considers to be your top priority: the negative belief or influence in your life that must be addressed in the session to bring the body back into balance.

We work with PSYCH-K to balance those negative beliefs and align the subconscious, conscious and super-conscious minds. Another round of testing leads us to the appropriate Body Brilliant session. We then move to the massage table and work with the deep polarity points to awaken the body's energy grid. Next we concentrate on the "armored band" of muscles and tissues for that session with somatic deep-tissue massage.

The massage work is followed by more polarity balancing. Each session focuses on one of these areas: the five elements (earth, water, fire, air, and ether), the chakras, the lymph, or the subtler nervous systems.

Further Reading

Clark, Dawn E. *Gifts for the Soul*. Houston, TX: Aarron Publishing, 1999–2001.

Clark, Dawn E. *The Gifts in Action*. Houston, TX: Aarron Publishing, 1999–2001.

Hanna, Thomas. *Somatics*. Reading, MA: Addison-Wesley Publishing, 1988.

Heller, Joseph and William A. Henkin. *BodyWise*. Oakland, CA: Wingbow Press, 1991.

Keleman, Stanley. *Emotional Anatomy*. Berkeley, CA: Center Press, 1985.

Lipton, Bruce H. *The Biology of Belief: Understanding the Power of Consciousness, Matter and Miracles*. Santa Rosa, CA: Mountain of Love/Elite Books, 2005.

Thie, John. *Touch for Health*. Camarillo, CA: Devorss & Co., 1973.

To like myself means to be, literally shameless, to be wanton in the pleasures of being inside a body ... the way I'd felt as a child before the world had interfered.

—Sallie Tisdale

4

BODY WISDOM

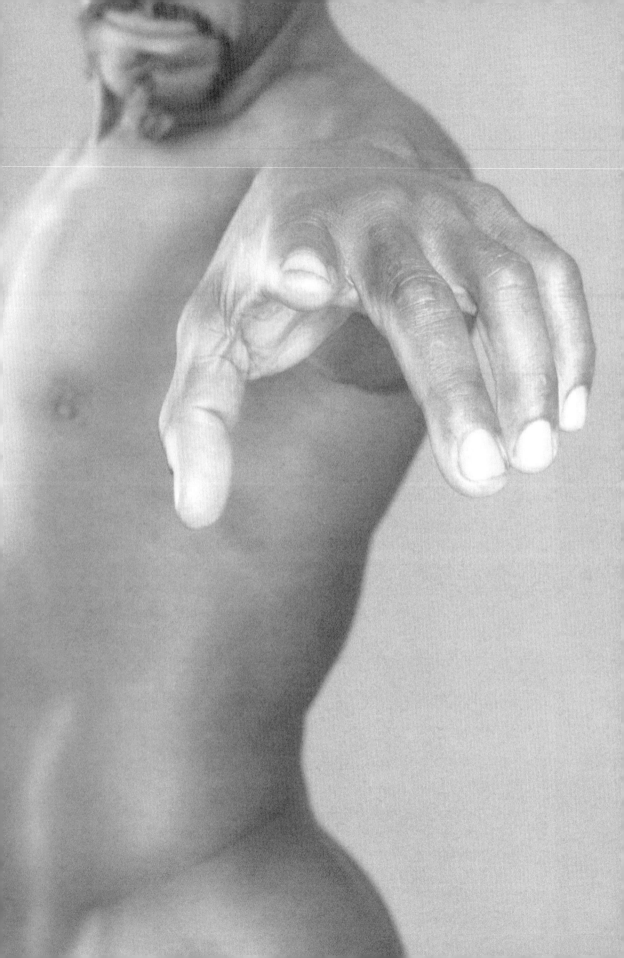

CHAPTER 20

Your Body Wisdom

*A cloud does not know why it moves in just such a direction
and at such a speed. It feels an impulse ... this is the place to go now.
But the sky knows the reasons and the patterns behind all clouds.*
—Richard Bach

ouston, Summer 1987: I was lying in bed praying, asking God for guidance. I wanted to know, "What can I do to know You better and Your will for me?" This had been my prayer for some weeks now. I'd been sober for six months by then. I'd just recently received my miraculous HIV-negative test results. I was burning with purpose. I knew, in spite of myself, some great good fortune had protected me from harm's way. I didn't (and still don't) think of God in the Christian way, but I felt preserved by someone for some purpose. I just didn't know what. Thus my regular calls to a higher power, the Great Spirit, the Tao.

What was this something I was destined to do? I'd felt a sense of it since I was a boy. For years I thought it was my simple vanity, just a lonely, misunderstood boy needing to feel important. But since my reprieve from the AIDS executioner stalking so many of my friends, I allowed myself to feel once again that deep longing inside me. But longing for what? It was just a vague sense that I had something special to do on this earth. So as I lay in bed that night repeating my call to know God better, I was hardly prepared to hear a voice, faint but clear, that said, "Quit eating meat."

I'd had hunches all my life; I often knew and understood things other people didn't seem to notice. But this was the first time those hunches had spoken to me in a voice I could hear in my head. Happily, I was in a place in life where I could even hear my inner voice and consider taking action on its advice. Intellectually, I knew many Hindus were vegetarian for spiritual reasons, but I never thought it was for me. Outside of corn and potatoes, I didn't care much for vegetables. But that night I decided to heed the voice and began an abstinence of all meats that would last more than six years.

We all have our own unique inner guidance, if we just listen for that voice. It's probably quite faint if you've spent more time attending to the world than listening for its wise advice. But it is there. In your quietest moments ask, "What feels best for me now?" The more carefully you listen, the more you will hear your inner voice and the louder it will speak through you. The more often you act on its advice the louder it will shout. Listening for that little voice is no different than learning from your body wisdom: complete trust in your body's internal knowledge yields positive—and still more possible—results.

My body wisdom is my guide through self-discovery. Some would call it intuition, inspiration, or divine intervention. It is the mouthpiece of that flickering light of truth in each human heart. It is the core knowledge that leads to greater understanding of myself: universal truth that is unique for me, expressed through that little voice deep within my mind. It was my body wisdom that spoke to me that night and said, "Quit eating meat." It was my body wisdom that spoke to me that day as I stood in line at Whole Foods Market, holding a pamphlet on massage therapy, telling me, "You can do this." I have never regretted heeding the voice's advice.

I believe that by heeding the voice's advice to start a lacto-ovo vegetarian diet (I still ate milk, cheese, and eggs), I was able to hear the voice speak to me even louder at Whole Foods Market. Learning to cook and enjoy a healthy vegetarian cuisine paved the way for me to join David Arpin, Mikel Reper, and Craig Ann in opening The Enchanted Garden. Just by taking the voice's first advice I was able to open one door after another. Not all of these "opportunities" led to smiley faces and happy endings. But following my inner compass took me on a continually deeper and richer journey. As the writer and spiritual teacher Alan Cohen says, "Life is like photography. We use the negative to develop." I have learned to love it all.

As a young man I was active in the Christian church. Once I realized being gay was my destiny and not a passing curiosity, I went through a mild depression (it was the 1970s; we were all finding ourselves). When the depression lifted I deeply understood, I knew: God created me this way, a gay man, and I was not a mistake or a sin.

Needless to say, my interpretation of God's purpose was not the same as that of the church. In those days homosexuals were considered intrinsically evil. So I walked away from the Christian church, confident that its judgments were wrong about me. It was many years before I separated the truth of "who Jesus is" from the churches that bear his name. By accepting my homosexuality I chose the margins of our society. I was forced to dig deeply within myself in order to find my own truth, that mystical fire that burns within each of us.

So how does one sense body wisdom? In the late 1980s, my good friend and fellow spiritual seeker J. D. and I joined a weekly meditation group led by Miles Glaspy. Week after week, for many years, I walked through the back gate, past the pool and the grape arbor, to climb the steps to Miles's place. Seven or eight of us fit snugly into his small attic office to plumb the depths of awareness demonstrated by Jean Huston's *The Possible Human* and *The Search for the Beloved*, *The Grief Recovery Handbook* by John James and Russell Friedman, and Japanese breathing techniques. In so doing we explored our own edges and our own possibilities.

I adapted the following visualization for sensing body wisdom from *The Possible Human*. I've had some extraordinary experiences with clients using the "Sensing Your Body Wisdom" meditation, as Suzie's story attests:

Suzie J. was trying to conceive. She and her husband had tried everything possible. Fertility clinics and drugs alone had failed to produce the pregnancy they wanted. Suzie added massage and acupuncture to enhance the work they were already doing with their doctors. Both Suzie and her husband attended a day of spiritual practice I held at Lake Livingston. It was a day of movement: Tai chi and yoga. It was also a day of meditations: guided, walking, sitting, and chanting. I led the "Sensing Your Body Wisdom" guided meditation after lunch. Foolish planning on my part! All but one person was dozing by the end of the meditation. At the break Suzie apologized for napping and asked if we could do the meditation again in a private session.

On her next visit to my office she lay on the table with my hands cradled under her head. I led her through the relaxation. As she met and talked with her Body Wisdom she began to cry. Her breathing choked as her tears rolled down her face. I guided her to relax into her feeling and open to it as much as possible. After some moments her breathing calmed and the tears stopped. I continued the meditation. When Suzie came out of the trance she told me what her Body Wisdom had shared. She had asked her Body Wisdom, "What can I do to get pregnant?" Her Body Wisdom reminded her of the pain and trauma of losing her virginity. She began to cry at the memory of it. Her Body Wisdom showed her how she had stifled her sexual vitality because of that traumatic event. She also felt the pain of living her adult life without enjoying her sexuality, which caused her to cry more.

Suzie was pregnant in a few months. Who can say what finally led to the successful pregnancy? Suzie and her husband were doing so much to support her body in conceiving. But Suzie firmly believes that meeting her Body Wisdom and releasing the trauma that blocked her sexual vitality played a pivotal role in her pregnancy.

Having seen the power of my own body wisdom, I agree with Suzie's conclusion.

There are several exercises and techniques that promote sensing one's Body Wisdom, such as structural massage (described in Chapters Eight and Nineteen), aromatherapy baths and most importantly, meditation: sitting, standing, alone or as part of a group. The following guided visualization works best if you can relax into a trance. Albert Einstein commented that, "Imagination is everything. It is the key to coming attractions." In a group setting one person is the narrator. If you are alone it is best to record it ahead of time in your own voice. Then sit back and listen to it without the interruptions of reading it piecemeal.

- Sit comfortably with your spine erect. Allow your eyes to close. Take several slow, deep breaths: one for body, one for heart, one for mind, one for spirit …

- In your mind's eye see yourself walking along a beach. It is twilight. Notice the sensations: the feel of the sand under your feet and the wind caressing your skin, the colors of sky and water, the sounds of birds and waves, the tastes and smells as you breathe in the ocean air.

- You approach a mountainous sand dune. Feel the exertion of climbing; it is steep and slow going. For each step up the dune you slip some backward as the sands fall beneath your feet. You lean into the angle of your climb. Your muscles strain with the effort, your chest heaves with each breath. You stop to rest for a moment. Turn to survey the night sky. There is no light except for the stars above you. You notice that the constellations, crystal clear and huge, have a peculiar angle. You name them easily, though you had forgotten their names long ago. Return to your vigorous climb.

- When you reach the top of the dune you see a stone building. As you walk up to it, still breathing hard, two doors slide open silently. Feeling totally safe you walk into the inner chamber. The doors close behind you as the small room glows with a purple light. You notice how the light affects your breath, your mood, and your body. The room begins to drop slowly into the earth. As you drop deeper into the earth the color changes to indigo. Notice how the change of color affects your body, your mood, and your thoughts. As the room drops deeper the colors change slowly from indigo, to blue, to green, to yellow, to orange, and, finally, red. The elevator stops and the doors open.

- Enter a long hallway that descends deeper still into the earth. Ancient symbols are chiseled onto stone walls. With your fingertips feel the secrets spelled out before you, in languages long forgotten. As you walk you are surprised by how much you begin to understand the hieroglyphs. You have a deeper wisdom than your waking mind allows.

- The hallway splits in two directions. One leads farther down into the earth. The other leads to a door. Turning to the door you read the runes that say Body Wisdom, your body wisdom. Open the door and enter. Stop and wonder at the vast library you see before you. Mezzanines rise above an open floor studded with tables and chairs for reading. Sculptures of atoms, cells, solar systems, and body organs are beautifully lit throughout. In the center of the room you see a being. While walking toward this being you stop to open a book. Surprised, you see multi-dimensional pictographs of truths, hallucinogenic in their vividness and clarity. Realize that this library, deep within your own consciousness, contains all the secrets of the universe.

- Recognize the being as your body wisdom. Smoking incense adds spice and mystery to the seated figure. You sense a deep peace with this presence. Approach and take a seat. Gaze into those wise eyes. Ask, "What do I need to know to love my life?" You listen intently for all that is revealed to you. You realize a few minutes of this streaming consciousness are equal to hours upon hours of your regular thinking time. You soak up the wisdom granted to you. As the stream of consciousness slows to a stop you sit quietly savoring the enormity of this gift. In gratitude you ask, "What can I do for you?" and listen once again for the reply. Gazing into the wise eyes you feel a healing light spread through your body. All your aches and pains disappear. All your fears and doubts leave you. You know the certainty of trust. You know your rightful place in the cosmic order.

• Knowing this visit is finished you stand, thanking your body wisdom once again. Understand you are to visit the library again. It is always here for you to study the truths that you seek. Exit through the door back into the chiseled hallway. Climbing toward the elevator your fingers once again trace the ancient symbols of the walls. Like reading Braille you now know what they mean. Snatches of mathematics, chemistry, metaphysics, and alchemy flood your thoughts as you trail upward to the elevator. The doors open to a vermillion red glow. Enter into the inner chamber. Sense once again how the color affects your thoughts and mood. The room climbs toward the earth's surface showering you with the colors of the rainbow as you rise: orange, yellow, green, blue, indigo, and purple. Finally the room fills with a golden light that permeates your every cell. The doors slowly open. Look out over the horizon. Breathe in the crisp morning air of a new dawn.

FURTHER READING

Hicks, Jerry, and Esther Hicks. *A New Beginning I: Handbook for Joyous Survival.* San Antonio, TX: Abraham-Hicks Publications, 2002.

Houston, Jean. *The Possible Human.* Los Angeles: J. Tarcher, 1982.

Huston, Jean. *The Search for The Beloved.* Los Angeles: J. Tarcher, 1987.

Visit www.BodyBrillianceBook.com to download your free written copy of these exercises.

Sit near a tree, a brook, a rock. Set aside your intellect.
Let the natural flow of the universe course
through your being and harmonize your soul.
Let it draw you into an eternal sense
of time and flow ...

—Ram Dass

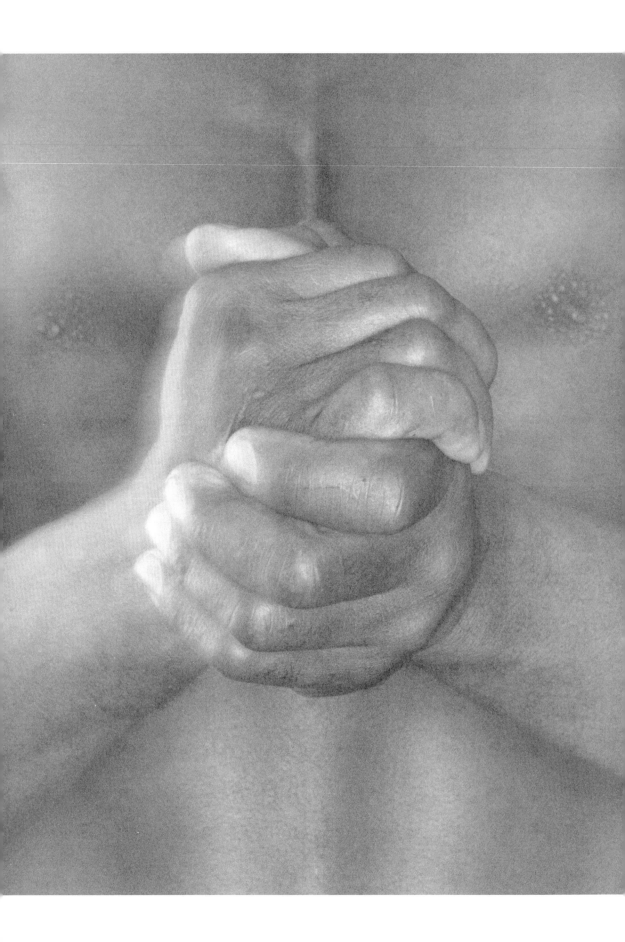

Sitting Meditation

The key to this meditation is simple: you focus on the sensations of your body as you sit. When you notice yourself thinking, which you will (it's what the mind is designed to do), gently return your attention to any of the sensations of your body. The skill of meditation is to consistently focus our attention in the present. The sensations of our body always happen in the present moment. When we focus our attention to those sensations we automatically tune to the present moment.

- Sit comfortably cross-legged on the floor with your spine straight. Placing a cushion just under your sitz bones (the bones of your pelvis you actually sit on) lifts your spine. It helps you to sit in peace and quiet. Turn off all the distractions you can—telephones, TV, music, kids. Gently close your eyes.

- Turn your attention to your feet and sense everything you can. Feel any pressure from the ground, your socks? Sense your skin and the feel of air or fabric on it. Do you have a sense of temperature? Of vibration? When you notice yourself thinking, gently bring your attention back to your body.

- Move your attention to your calves, hips, and thighs. Sense the weight of your body pressing on the floor. Sense your skin and the feel of air or fabric on it. Do you have a sense of temperature? Of vibration? When you begin thinking, gently return your attention to your body.

- Move your attention to your belly. Soften your belly. Let your muscles and guts relax. Sense your skin and the feel of air or fabric on it. Do you have a sense of temperature? Of vibration? When you notice yourself thinking, gently return your attention to your body.

- Move your attention to your back. Sense the muscles and bones that hold you erect as you sit. If there is tension or pain in your back turn your attention to it and take a deep breath. Direct your breath to the tension. The movement and attention of your breath may soften that tension. Sense your skin and the feel of air or fabric on it. Do you have a sense of temperature? Of vibration? When you notice yourself thinking, gently bring your attention back to your body.

- Move your attention to your breath. Notice the rising and falling of your chest. Sense the air moving in and out of your chest. Sense your skin and the feel of air or fabric on it. Do you have a sense of temperature? Of vibration? When you notice yourself thinking, gently bring your attention back to your body.

- Move your attention to your neck and head. Sense the movement of air across your upper lip as you breathe. Feel the movement of air through your nose and throat. Notice any aromas or tastes you experience. Sense your skin and hair. Do you have a sense of temperature? Of vibration? When you notice yourself thinking, gently bring your attention back to your body.

- Return to the sensations of your feet and move back up your body to the head and neck. Initially sit for twenty minutes. As you are comfortable, increase your sitting time by ten-minute increments until you can sit for one hour.

*This is the first, wildest, and wisest thing
I know, that the soul exists, and that it is
built entirely out of attention.*

—Mary Oliver

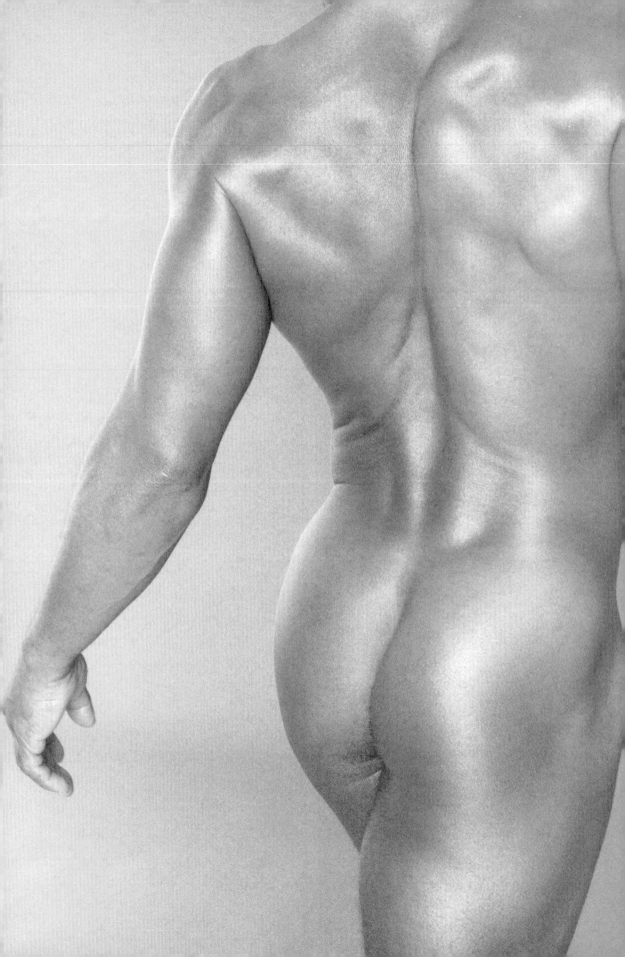

Standing Meditation

- Ground yourself by standing with your feet hips-width apart. Relax your body and feel your feet on the floor. Feel the actual sensations of pressure, temperature, or vibration as you stand. Notice how your body weight is distributed upon your feet. Now raise one leg and stomp down. Raise the other leg and stomp. Gently bend your knees and notice the change in sensations in your body. Repeat the stomp and knee bend three more times. Notice the sensations of your stance after each stomp.

- Place the heels of your hands just above the knees. Drop your tailbone. You should feel your whole upper body pressing down onto the heels of your hands. Look over a shoulder and exhale. As you breathe out make a guttural sound in your throat. Visualize energy moving from the tip of your tailbone, up along the spine, and out the throat. Look over the other shoulder and repeat the order. This exercise increases vitality.

- Stand upright. Wobble your body a bit until you find a comfortable stance. Close your eyes three-quarters of the way. Let your breath find its natural rhythm. Turn your attention to your feet. Notice the sensations of standing: your feet on the ground, the feeling of shoes or socks on your feet. Do you have a sense of temperature? Of vibration? Of pressure? When you notice yourself thinking, return your attention to your body.

- Turn your attention to your legs, hips, groin, and genitals. Notice the sensations of your legs meeting the pelvis and the weight of your upper body. Do you have a sense of temperature? Of vibration? Of pressure? When you notice yourself thinking, gently bring your attention back to your body.

- Move your attention to your belly. Soften your belly. Let your muscles and guts relax. Sense your skin and the feel of air or fabric on it. Do you have a sense of temperature? Of vibration? Of pressure? When you notice yourself thinking, gently bring your attention back to your body.

- Sense your back and the muscles and bones that hold you erect as you stand. If there is tension or pain in your back turn your attention to it and take a deep breath. Direct your breath to the tension. The movement and attention of your breath will often soften that tension. Sense your skin and the feel of air or fabric on it. Do you have a sense of temperature? Of vibration? When you notice yourself thinking, gently bring your attention back to your body.

- Move your attention to your breath. Notice the rising and falling of your chest. Sense the air moving in and out of your chest. Sense your skin and the feel of air or fabric on it. Do you have a sense of temperature? Of vibration? Of pressure? When you notice yourself thinking, gently bring your attention back to your body.

- Move your attention to your neck and head. Sense the movement of air across your upper lip as you breathe. Feel the movement of air through your nose and throat. Notice any aromas or tastes you have. Sense your skin and hair. Do you have a sense of temperature? Of vibration? When you notice yourself thinking, gently bring your attention back to your body.

- Return to the sensations of your feet, standing, and repeat the sensory scan of your body for your standing meditation.

Our bodies are our gardens,
to which our wills are gardeners.

—Othello

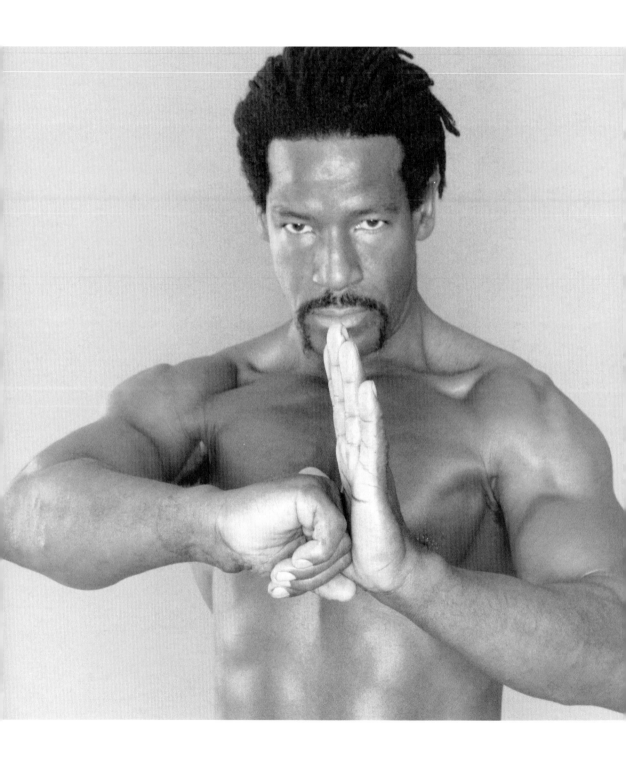

Structural Massage

You will be able to do most of the exercises in this book by yourself or with a friend. However, deep-structural massage requires expert training and skill. You will have to find a deep-structural massage artist to experience the benefits available to your posture and your life. There are several ways to find a qualified therapist with presence. The best and easiest way is by word of mouth: a referral from someone you trust. The other way is to interview a therapist. Ask about his or her training and approach to the work. Most importantly, trust your own good sense.

I mentioned "presence" as a qualification: The ability to be present, to accept any and all emotions and experiences that could arise during a therapy session, creates a safe place for emotional, confidential work. Whether or not a therapist possesses presence is the first thing I consider when choosing a deep-tissue practitioner.

Some sources to help you locate deep-tissue bodyworkers in your area:

The Rolf Institute of Structural Integration
5055 Chaparral Ct. Suite 103
Boulder, CO 80301
Phone: (303), 449-5903, (800) 530-8875
Fax: (303) 449-5978

Hellerwork School of Structural Integration
PO Box 23730
San Diego, CA 92193-3730
Phone: (858) 279 1959
Fax: (858) 279 1989

Guild For Structural Integration
3107 28th St.
Boulder, CO 80301
Phone: (800) 447-0150

Lomi School Foundation and Psychotherapy Clinic
2455 Bennett Valley Road Suite C-218
Santa Rosa, CA 95404
Phone: (707) 579-0465
Fax: (707) 579-0560
www.zentherapy.org

Aromatherapy Bath

Aromatherapy refers to the use of essential oils extracted from plants which promote balancing and healing of the body, mind, heart, and soul. These oils are the most potent form of plant energy we have to work with. Most essential oils are extracted from their plants using steam distillation. Every essential oil has its own specific properties that affect the different aspects of our lives.

A hot aromatherapy bath after a deep-tissue massage, including bath salts and vinegar, helps the muscles to continue to flush out lactic acid   and other toxins that have built up. It also helps the connective tissues to soften and stretch. The salts and vinegar help neutralize any static electricity in the system, while the essential oils help to ground and expand the consciousness as well as clear your energetic field.

Just as in making a fine soup, one needs to have an all-purpose base, which can then be amended. For my base I combine:

1 cup Dead Sea mineral salts

1 cup baking soda

1 cup apple cider vinegar.

Then I add twenty drops in total of any one or combination of these pure essential oils:

- Cedarwood

- Frankincense

- Myrrh

- Patchouli

- Vetiver.

Each of these oils represents the earth and promotes grounding. Vetiver is distilled from the roots of a tall, dense, aromatic grass originally grown in Southeast Asia, and the others come from types of wood. Myrrh, frankincense, and cedarwood also activate the psychic centers of the brain, adding an expansive edge to the sense of being grounded.

Visit www.BodyBrillianceBook.com to download your free written copy of more aromatherapy recipes.

*We all have a genuine intelligence that
is ripe with insight and compassion. Intelligence is
unearthed by consciously lived experiences and
not by the simple knowing of facts and symbols ...
I'm talking about how we conduct and use ourselves
in everyday life; standing, holding, yielding, embracing,
opening our eyes, taking a breath. It is in these prelimi-
nary actions that we can come to experience our intelligence and not just have an idea about it.*

—Richard Strozzi-Heckler

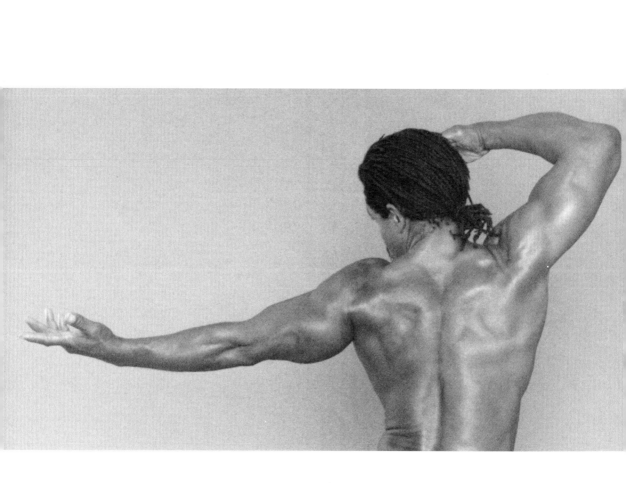

CHAPTER 21

Repetition Is the Key

We are what we repeatedly do.
Excellence, then, is not an act, but a habit.
—Aristotle

How can you best use this book? I'm reminded of the advice I received in a Chinese fortune cookie once, which wisely stated, "None of the secrets of success will work unless you do." My master plan for the Body Brilliance series is to:

- introduce you to body-centered principles and exercises for your life
- inspire you to practice these body-centered principles and exercises on a regular basis, trusting that your own practice will lead you to deeper truth and happiness
- encourage you to live your truth and happiness in the world.

The Body Brilliance series is divided into three books, encompassing the basic principles of a body-centered life and the five vital layers of intelligence (IQs).

This first book lays the foundations: the principles and exercises that maximize the life force in our bodies, our physical intelligence. I offer exercises in each section that help me to continually deepen my experience of myself, to seek the truth, to heal, and to enjoy my life.

The spiritual principles that inform the world's mystical traditions continue to inspire me to further exploration in the areas of touch, movement, sex, eating, breathing, speaking, thinking, and mystical activism. Although for simplicity's sake I will address each of these topics individually, remember that each falls into one of the five layers of vital intelligence. When integrated into a body-centered approach to living, the reward—to experience life without boundaries or distinctions—exceeds the benefits of pursuing any area alone.

Older dogs can learn new tricks, but mastering anything unfamiliar takes time, motivation, patience, and practice. Growing one's consciousness requires com-mitment and understanding of the learning process. Learning occurs in four stages:

- The unconscious stage of learning is clueless (we don't even know that we don't know).

- The awareness stage enables us to learn what we realize we don't know.

- The skill or fitness stage indicates a level of competency in learning, but we still have to remember to use our tools, especially under stress, or risk compromising our abilities.

- The mastery level represents intimate knowing; skills and principles are integrated so seamlessly into our character and response that they become part of our psyche.

The basic principles discussed in the Body Brilliance series will work for everyone if they choose to use them. In the expanse of human consciousness, including the 5,000 years of written history, there are an extraordinary number of exercises designed to improve health and happiness and to teach self-realization.

Yet each of us is unique with different interests and temperaments. I am sharing the exercises that work for me, a tall, gay man with a fulfilling career and a rewarding personal life. I have twenty-five-plus years of experience in asking questions and in sincerely listening for their answers. I know principles and exercises, but what I am sharing is not new. These principles are as old as the universe itself. My contribution is to organize them and speak them in plain English, in a way that you may understand them and use them in your everyday life.

Richard Bach says in *Illusions,* "We are all teachers, learners, doers." Socrates told his students to "question everything." There are many opinions and schools of thought that claim to be the way to truth. Mohandas Mahatma Gandhi said, "Only truth is God. I am a human being. Truth for me is changing every day. My commitment must be to truth, not to consistency."

Carlos Castañeda wrote a number of books about the teachings of Don Juan, a Mexican *curandero,* or medicine man. Don Juan put it this way:

> Look at every path closely and deliberately. Try it as many times as you think necessary. Then ask yourself and yourself alone one question. This question is one that only a very old man asks. My benefactor told me about it once when I was young and my blood was too vigorous for me to understand it. Now I do understand it. I will tell you what it is: Does this path have a heart? If it does, the path is good. If it doesn't, it is of no use.

I once interviewed Jacques Verduin, a somatic teacher, psychotherapist and bodyworker, who spoke of "getting people hooked, of seducing people to be curious about being alive." I love the idea of spiritual seduction. It's like the romantic stage of any relationship. I need that initial infatuation to start the momentum, to overcome the difficulties.

It is human nature to be creatures of habit. We drive the same way to work every day, we eat in the same few restaurants, we stand around in the same slouch, we use the same vocabulary and expressions when we talk, we hang with the same people. The habitual, minuscule movements of our bodies usually fly under the radar screens of our attention and are ignored until our muscles won't stretch any farther and the nerves contract in pain. Our breathing may have become so shallow or labored that the lungs are barely supplying oxygen to the heart and brain. After a while, our lives shrink to nothing more than repetitive patterns of movement—and those aren't usually very healthy.

What I hope the Body Brilliance series shows you is that whether you are an athlete or a couch potato, your habits can change from self-defeating to self-enriching. Maintaining a spiritual program is a lifelong challenge, and everyone must find the principles and teachers that inspire him or her to commit to a systematic, nononsense, regular practice. But revitalizing your mind and body is joyous and rewarding work.

I use meditation as a metaphor to live my life. In the sensing your body exercises (Chapter Twenty) I directed you to focus your attention on some of the many different sensations of your body as you sat. When your mind wandered I asked that you simply, and gently, bring your attention back to your body. Allow your body's sensations to anchor your attention. And when your mind wanders, again and again, just keep coming back to your body, over and over. That is the art and skill of learning attention. Eventually, with regular practice we develop unshakable focus.

I have a set of somatic exercises that I enjoy for growing consciousness. Some periods of my life I actively pursue them, other periods they wane. Some months my diet is good, and some years I practice my yoga faithfully. Sometimes that focus fades, and I switch to strengthening my body or attending to my swaying posture. But I keep coming back to pick them up. Year after year I come back to the exercises that I know help me feel better.

The first step in peaking our vital intelligences is to recognize who and where we are: a radical acceptance of the habits and the repeated patterns, large and small, which govern our lives. The Swiss psychiatrist Carl Jung said, "The greatest sin is to be unconscious." Yet most of us go through life that way.

The second step to peaking our Intelligences is deciding who we want to be and where we want to go with our lives. What do we want more of—more life, more love, more consciousness, more money, more truth—and how much is enough? What is the best path to achieve our desires? And how do we prepare for the journey? This is the point when our body wisdom guides us with its little voice, telling those who will listen how to feel better, love better, live better, and be better.

The third step is simply to pay attention: to be mindful of our habits and how best to improve them. This step requires infinite patience. I am reminded of a speech given by Hester Lampert-Hill from Beth Israel Hospital in Boston. She is a social worker for cancer patients, survivors and their families.

In her speech, Lampert-Hill talked about the paradox of Sisyphus. Sisyphus was king of the Greek city of Corinth and something of a trickster. His too-clever pranks offended the gods, however, who condemned Sisyphus to roll a giant boulder up a hill. Just as he would reach the top, the boulder would roll back down again. His task incomplete, Sisyphus would start over, day after day, for eternity. Worse than the grueling physical effort was the knowledge that each attempt to succeed was futile.

Still, Sisyphus gave that boulder another go every day, and for his persistence Lampert-Hill called him a hero. She described all those quiet people who battle tremendous odds daily, particularly cancer social workers, as unsung heroes. They work ceaselessly to boast of small successes in the face of crushing tragedies. And yet like Sisyphus they soldier on, offering help, comfort, and courage to those who need it most.

The third step of growing consciousness demands that each of us be heroes, often unrecognized, attending to our bodies, hearts, and minds in the light of day and the dark of night. Sometimes the task seems futile and overwhelming, as it may take a lifetime to dissolve old patterns of fear. It takes attention. But the effort is *worth* the pain. Allow your longing for the truth to strengthen your commitment, and let us journey together for a while to see what we can learn and teach each other.

As a kid I used to watch the old Ed Sullivan variety show. He would often host a plate spinner. A man, dressed in black slacks and a colorful shirt, would stand before a number of metal poles cut to different heights. To the strains of dramatic music he would place a white plate atop a pole, balance it, and spin it. As long as the plate continued to spin, it remained balanced on the pole. The man would place more and more spinning plates on top of more poles. He would, however, have to go back to re-spin plates as they began to slow down and wobble. His trick and skill was to keep as many plates spinning as possible without one crashing to the floor and breaking. It was an impressive trick.

Living a somatic life, living through your body—or any spiritual life path—is a bit like spinning plates. At this first level of intelligence there is a plate for good posture, and there are plates for flexibility, strength, and grace. Add good attention to each of these and there is the potential to have many plates spinning simultaneously. We haven't yet added the plates for the other four layers of intelligence— or for good breathing, eating, sacred sex, thinking, listening, honesty, service, or vital energy.

In the end we learn to spin plates like a master juggler. But sometimes the plates wobble and stop, or fall and break. The key to success here is, when it feels good, pick up another plate and spin again. Keep playing.

I try not to compare myself to others. There will always be people who stand better and taller, are more flexible (a lot, actually), are stronger, more fit, or thinner, or more graceful. I try every day to make the very best of what life offers to me. I make peace with my limitations and my best efforts. I keep in mind the words of the mystic Sufi poet Jalaluddin Rumi:

> *Come, Come, whoever you are!*
> *Wanderer, worshiper, lover of leaving.*
> *Come, Come.*

This is not a caravan of despair.
It doesn't matter if you've broken your vow a thousand times, still
Come, and yet again come.
—*The Illuminated Rumi*
(translated by Coleman Barks)

I am not teaching enlightenment per se. Oh, in the folly of my youth I liked to think I would be enlightened by the time of my death. In my travels, both inner and outer, I have glimpsed the tremendous attention required to wake up and live an enlightened life. I do not have the motivation this time around for enlightenment. I do have the inspiration and commitment to grow consciousness, to peak my intelligences, to practice truth, to be healthy in body, heart, mind, and soul, to be happy, to live a life meaningful to me and to share it with the world I live in. Albert Camus said, "But what is happiness except the simple harmony between man and the life he leads.?"

I expect you have a similar commitment. You exercise it every time you seek to do good in your world, to understand who you are, and how you affect the people around you. You do it every time you ask, "What is the meaning of my life?" You demonstrate it by reading books like this one.

Tomales, California, December 1994: I zipped along California's scenic coastal Highway 1. Sheila, sitting next to me, encouraged me to cut the Porsche loose, but I was afraid. I'd never driven a car of this power (or this price tag). I was overly cautious so as not to wreck her car. The engine purred as I punched the accelerator, and we thrilled as the hairpin turns flew by.

I laughed as the Porsche squealed to a stop at the Tomales Bakery. Stocked with tasty treats, we sped to Dillon Beach. Seventeen of us were piling into a four-bedroom house perched above the Pacific Ocean, residing together for the last weekend of our Lomi training. We had rented this house back in July for our weeklong intensive. We'd had so much fun that we decided to rent it again for our final weekend together.

Sheila and I, as planned, were the first to arrive. We opened the house to the cold December breezes and staked our claim on a small bedroom with two twin beds. Snacking on pastries we spot-cleaned the house and unpacked the first run of groceries.

Things in order, I walked down the steep switchback road to the beach. I had come to love this stretch of coastline and my long walks in the cold wind. The sun warmed my face as my hands snuggled in my coat. I marveled that the northern Pacific wind, even in winter, was so delicious. I strolled along, anticipating the weekend slumber party and our last two days with Richard and Robert.

The Lomi School was proving to be the best gift I've given myself in quite a few years and, by far, the best therapy. This was the tenth month of our training. I felt a world of difference from that first weekend back in March. I had paid my debt down by thousands of dollars—a long way to go, but a good start. My depression had lifted. I still felt pangs of regret over the closing of The Enchanted Garden and the sting of Michael's death. Waves of grief and sadness still broke over my heart. But they passed. My easy smile and laugh were frequent visitors. My work thrived.

Even some long-cherished dreams were coming true. My friend Nancy Winters and I had talked long and often of an advanced training program for massage therapists. So, inspired by my training at the Lomi School, by Robert and Richard, and fueled by their stories of Randolph Stone and some new techniques, I offered a thirty-two-hour polarity therapy class. Twelve eager students enrolled. I incorporated movement and meditation into the training along with the energy bodywork. The group's enthusiasm for the work and the seminar were deeply satisfying. Nancy and I arranged for a percentage split of the class profits, so I made some good money as well. Starting on the downside, 1994 had turned around.

On our last night at the beach house, Molly cooked dinner. The whole class showed up to celebrate. We sat crowded around the living room eating African ground-nut stew the traditional way, scooping it with our hands. We wolfed down the delicious meal, laughing together, rehashing the year's events. Everyone had a favorite tale to remember. Our Israeli chiropractor, Nir, slipped a cassette tape of the Gypsy Kings into the stereo and turned up the volume. Furniture was shoved back and the dancing began. I grabbed a scarf as Erika and I improvised a flamenco.

Hot and sweaty after much dancing, I stepped out into the night. I walked farther up the hill, draping the scarf around my shoulders for warmth. The ocean was barely visible far below in the starlight. Facing the crash of the waves I squatted down to rest on my heels and watched my breath steaming in the cold air. It took a minute to register, but I felt something. It felt good, really good. Something lost long ago and just now found. I felt alive, excited, and very simply happy. This year was proving to be my best year yet. The sound of music and laughter carried up the hill. I shivered with a chill as my wet body cooled.

I sat for a long while, savoring my happiness. A few minutes later I wandered back through the starlight to rejoin the dancing.

Make the journey to better health and vitality. Shine through the peaking of your vital intelligences. Dance and sing and enjoy life to the fullest.

Be brilliant.

... Do not now seek the answers, which cannot be given you because you would not be able to live them. And the point is, to live everything. Live the questions now. Perhaps you will gradually, without noticing it, live along some distant day into the answer.

Resolve to be always beginning—to be a beginner!

—Rainer Maria Rilke

Appendix:
The Body Brilliance Kata

Kata means "form." In martial arts practice, a kata is a short series of movements which are repeated, over and over, until they are second nature. And once they are eventually mastered, they are seamlessly integrated into one's essential nature. The Body Brilliance kata works through all five layers of our vital intelligence; physical, emotional, mental, moral, and spiritual, to peak and balance them. I repeat this exercise kata five to six days a week, rotating between Kata-Day 1, which focuses on the joints and their mobility; and Kata-Day 2, which on focuses on muscle flexibility. It takes me about 45 minutes per session. If I'm low on time I shorten my routine by choosing a few exercises from each category: Tai chi, joints drills or flexibility, strength, and I always include the Five Tibetans. When I have longer to indulge myself with the Kata, I lengthen some of the exercises, especially the yoga poses on day 2. I also sit longer for my meditation time.

I often go to a quiet grove near Allen Parkway, a stretch of park near my house, to enjoy the beauty of nature while I kata. It's a treat to glide through the Tai chi Five Elements outdoors. It's a real thrill to do a headstand against a 70 foot pine tree and watch the joggers run by (upside-down).

Committing to the Body Brilliance Kata (or any body/mind/spirit practice) is part of the necessary and systematic effort needed to change, evolve, and grow. As with every path, you will see spurts of dramatic growth, alternating with periods of much more subtle change. It's your body/mind/spirit adapting to your new altitude of evolution. You are integrating all the subtle shifts that continue to draw you up your spiral of personal and spiritual growth. Choose your perfect life. And choose to let it be fun and easy. Be you. Make it so.

Body Brilliance Kata: Day 1

1. Tai Chi Five Elements—Clockwise turn (Left foot back in Heaven and Earth)

2. Joint Mobility Drills—***

   a. Ankle Circles

   b. Knee Circles

   c. Hindu Squats

   d. Hula Hoop

   e. Belly Dance

   f. The Cossack

   g. Split Switches

   h. Shoulder Circles

   i. Elbow Circles

   j. Wrist Rotations

   k. Fist Exercise

   l. The Egyptian

   m. Arm Circles

   n. Three Plane Neck Movements

   o. Cat/Cow Spinal Stretch

   p. Spine Rotation

3. Conscious Calisthenics—

   a. Push Ups

   b. Bench Dips

   c. Back and Leg Lifts

   d. Crunches

4. Five Tibetans—The Dervish is Counter-Clockwise

5. Relaxation Visualization—Five to ten minutes

6. Meditation— Five to ten minutes

***Visit www.BodyBrillianceBook.com to download your free written copy of these exercises.

Body Brilliance Kata: Day 2

1. Tai Chi—Counter Clockwise (Right foot back in Heaven and Earth)
2. Conscious Calisthenics—
   a. Diamond Push Ups
   b. Bench Dips
   c. Ins and Outs, or Bicycles
   d. Walking Lunges
3. Five Tibetans—Dervish—Clockwise
4. Flexibility—You'll be plenty warmed up after those Tibetans
   a. Easy Toe Touch
   b. Hamstring Stretch/IT Band Stretch
   c. Triangle (or Right Angle/or Reverse Triangle)
   d. The Tree, (or The Dancer/or The Eagle)
   e. Standing Head to Knee/(or Forward Fold/or The Plier)
   f. The Camel
   g. Shoulder Stand
   h. The Plow
   i. The Fish
   j. The Cobra
   k. The Locust
   l. The Bow
   m. Headstand
   n. Child's Pose
   o. Lying Down Spinal Twist
   p. Corpse Pose
5. Relaxation Visualization
6. Meditation

Visit www.BodyBrillianceBook.com to download your free written copy of these exercises.

Index

Bibliography

Aristotle. *Ethics*. Bath, England: The Folio Society, 2003.

"Albert Einstein." Wikipedia, the free encyclopedia. Available online at http://www.wikipedia.org/wiki/Albert_Einstein. Downloaded Feb. 27, 2006.

Barks, Coleman. *The Illuminated Rumi*. New York: Broadway Books, 1997.

Baum, Alisa. "Is Yoga Enough to Keep You Fit?" *Yoga Journal*. Sept./Oct. 2002.

Berenbaum, Michael. *The World Must Know: The History of the Holocaust*. Boston: Little, Brown and Co., 1993.

Budilovsky, Joan, and Eve Adamson. *The Complete Idiot's Guide to Yoga*. New York: Alpha Books, 1998.

Canfield, Jack. *The Power of Focus*. Deerfield Beach, FL: Health Communications, 2000.

Choudhury, Bikram, and Bonnie Jones Reynolds. *Bikram's Beginning Yoga Class*. New York: Tarcher/Putnam Books, 1978.

Chungliang Al Huang. *Quantum Soup*. New York: E. Dutton, 1983.

----------. *Tiger Return to Mountain*. Moab, UT: Real People Press, 1973.

Clark, Dawn E. *Gifts for the Soul*. Houston, TX: Aarron Publishing, 1999–2001.

----------. *The Gifts in Action*. Houston, TX: Aarron Publishing, 1999–2001.

Csikszentmihalyi, Mihaly. *Flow: The Psychology of Optimal Experience*. New York: Harper & Row, 1990: 2.

Davis, Kenneth C. *Don't Know Much About Mythology*. New York: HarperCollins, 2005.

Deuster, Patricia A., ed. *The Navy SEAL Physical Fitness Guide*. Old Saybrook, CT: Konecky & Konecky, 1997.

Easwaran, Eknath. *Gandhi the Man*. Petaluma, CA: Nilgiri Press, 1978.

Fadiman, James, and Robert Frager. *Personality and Personal Growth*. New York: Harper & Row, 1976.

Frankl, Viktor. *Man's Search for Meaning*. New York: Pocket Books, 1997.

Gagnon, Michelle. "Strong Abs for Life." *Yoga Journal*. Jan./Feb. 2003.

Gardner, Howard. *Frames of Mind: The Theory of Multiple Intelligences.* New York: BasicBooks, 1993.

Goleman, Daniel. *Emotional Intelligence: Why It Can Matter More Than IQ.* New York: Bantam Books, 1995.

Gudmestad, Julie. "Better Posture 101." *Yoga Journal.* October 2004.

Hanna, Thomas. *Somatics.* Reading, MA: Addison-Wesley Publishing, 1988.

Harvey, Andrew. *The Essential Gay Mystics.* Edison, NJ: Castle Books, 1997.

------------------. *The Way of Passion: A Celebration of Rumi.* Berkeley, CA.: Frog Ltd. Publishing, 1994.

Hawkins, David R. *Power vs. Force: The Anatomy of Consciousness.* Sedona, AZ: Veritas, 1995.

Heller, Joseph, and William A. Henkin. *BodyWise.* Oakland, CA: Wingbow Press, 1991.

Hicks, Jerry, and Esther Hicks. *A New Beginning I: Handbook for Joyous Survival.* San Antonio, TX: Abraham-Hicks Publications, 2002.

"HoloBarre System, The." Available online at www.users.interport.net/p/h/ physical/. Downloaded Aug. 8, 2004.

Huston, Jean. *The Possible Human.* Los Angeles: J. Tarcher, 1982.

----------. *The Search for The Beloved.* Los Angeles: J. Tarcher, 1987.

Hutchins, Kam. "An Interview with Ken Hutchins: Developer of the SuperSlow® Exercise Protocol." Available online at www.superslow.com/features/interview. htm. Downloaded Aug. 8, 2004.

Johansen, Greg, and Ron Kurtz. *Grace Unfolding.* New York: Bell Tower, 1991.

Kelder, Peter. *Ancient Secrets of the Fountain of Youth: Book 1.* New York: Doubleday, 1998.

Keleman, Stanley. *Emotional Anatomy.* Berkeley, CA: Center Press, 1985.

Kilham, Christopher S. *The Five Tibetans.* Rochester, VT: Healing Arts Press, 1994.

Knittel, Linda. "Deep Impact." *Yoga Journal.* July/August 2002.

Koontz, Dean. *From the Corner of His Eye.* New York: Bantam Books, 2001.

Kornfield, Jack. *A Path with Heart.* New York: Bantam Books, 1993.

Kreahling, Lorraine. "New Thoughts About When Not to Stretch." *The New York Times,* April 27, 2004.

Leonard, George. "Towards a Balanced Way." *The Lomi Papers*. Mill Valley, CA: The Lomi School, 1979.

Lidell, Lucy, with Narayani and Giris Rabinovitch. *The Sivananda Companion to Yoga*. London: Gaia Books, 1983.

Lipton, Bruce H. *The Biology of Belief: Understanding the Power of Consciousness, Matter and Miracles*. Santa Rosa, CA: Mountain of Love/Elite Books, 2005.

Loehr, Jim, and Tony Schwartz. *The Power of Full Engagement: Managing Energy, Not Time, Is the Key to High Performance and Personal Renewal*. New York: Free Press, 2003.

Meadow, Herb. "Nine Lives." *Kung Fu*. Warner Brothers: Burbank, CA, 1972.

Mitchell, Stephen. *Tao Te Ching*. New York: Harper & Row, 1988.

Muir, Charles and Caroline Muir. *Tantra: The Art of Conscious Loving*. San Francisco: Mercury House, 1989.

Nickerson, Nancy. "My Hero Project: Wilma Rudolph." Available online at www.myhero.com/myhero/hero.asp?hero=wilmaRudolph. Downloaded July 31, 2004.

Oschman, James L., and Nora Oschman. "Somatic Recall," part 1. *Massage Therapy Journal*, Summer 1995.

------------. "Somatic Recall," part 2. *Massage Therapy Journal*, Autumn 1995.

Perfetti, Ron. "Tíai Chi Ch'uan." Available online at www.ronperfetti.com/index.html. Downloaded Aug. 29, 2004.

Perls, Fritz. *Gestalt Therapy: Excitement and Growth in the Human Personality*. 1951.

Popkin, Richard H., and Avrum Stroll. *Philosophy Made Simple*. Garden City, NY: Doubleday & Co., 1956.

Prasad, Rama, and Caroline Robertson. "The Five Tibetans: Easy Energizing Exercises." Available online at: www.ayurvedaelements.com/img/five.pdf. Downloaded Sept. 4, 2004.

Reich, Wilhelm. *Character Analysis*. New York: Noonday Press, 1962.

Richman, Michael. "Scientist Albert Einstein: Persistence Made Him One of the Greatest Thinkers." *Investor's Business Daily*, Aug. 6, 2001. Available online at www.investors.com. Downloaded Feb. 27, 2006.

Rolf, Ida P. *Rolfing*. Rochester, VT: Healing Arts Press, 1989.

Seligman, Martin. *Authentic Happiness.* New York: Free Press, 2002.

"Sir Isaac Newton." Available online at www.isaacnewton.utwente.ul/nieuw/sir_isaac_newton/SirIsaacNewton.htm Downloaded Jan. 2, 2005.

Stone, Randolph. *Polarity Therapy: The Complete Collected Works.* Reno, NV: CRCS Publications, 1986.

Strozzi-Heckler, Richard. "A Holy Curiosity." *Whole Earth Review.* Spring 1994.

Thie, John. *Touch for Health.* Camarillo, CA: Devorss & Co., 1973.

Tsatsouline, Pavel. *Relax into Stretch.* St. Paul, MN: Dragon Door Publishing, 2001.

Wilber, Ken. "Introduction to Integral Theory and Practice." Integral Naked 2003–2004. Available online at www.integralnaked.org. Downloaded January 2006.

Wing, R. L. *The Illustrated I Ching.* Garden City, NY: Dolphin Books, 1982.

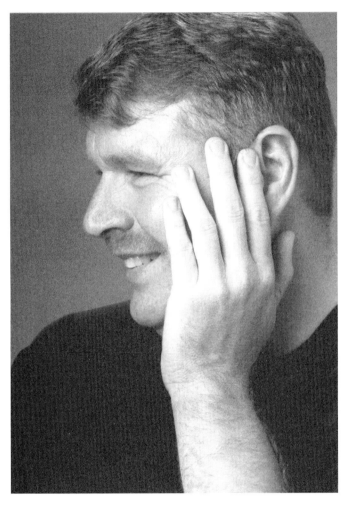

About the Author

Alan Davidson is a contributing author to *Healing the Heart of the World*, a compendium of essays by such authors as HRH Prince Charles, Caroline Myss, John Gray, Andrew Harvey, Naomi Judd, and Neale Donald Walsch. Alan, a Registered Massage Therapist since 1988, is the owner and director of Essential Touch Therapies in Houston, Texas. He has a bachelor's degree from the University of Houston–Downtown, with an emphasis on psychology, sociology, philosophy, and religion. Alan is fascinated with the intersection of bodywork, psychology, ritual, and spiritual practice. Having taught massage, meditation, yoga, and human transformation since 1990, he is currently on the teaching staff at NiaMoves Studio. Alan sums up his years of study with one wholehearted belief: "Life is for the fun of it!"

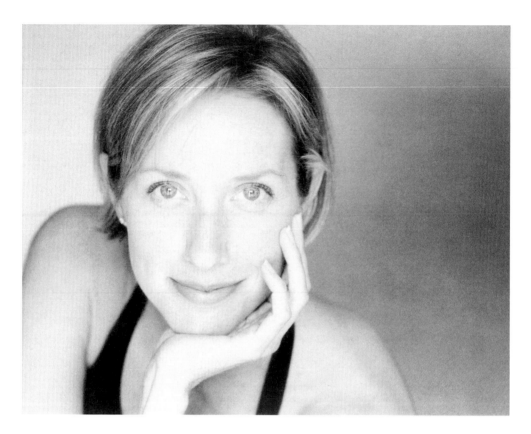

Victoria Davis, a Wisconsin native, has turned what she sees in the camera into an art form that's far-reaching in many ways. Her skillful artistry captures subtle but striking moments of beauty. Her unique ability to reveal the simple, natural optimism inherent in all her subjects sets her apart. Davis's signature is her use of natural lighting and her ability to capture "natural moments of spontaneity" in her photographs. Her most recent book, *Shakti: The Feminine Power of Yoga,* is a collection of stunning photographs celebrating the magnificence of the feminine power of yoga and has earned her rave reviews.